Get Intimate with Tantric Sex

This book is dedicated to my goddess, my Shakti, *who has brought me* ananda.

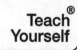
Teach® Yourself

Get Intimate with Tantric Sex

Paul Jenner

For UK order enquiries: please contact Bookpoint Ltd,
130 Milton Park, Abingdon, Oxon OX14 4SB.
Telephone: +44 (0) 1235 827720. Fax: +44 (0) 1235 400454.
Lines are open 09.00–17.00, Monday to Saturday, with a 24-hour
message answering service. Details about our titles and how to
order are available at www.teachyourself.com

Long renowned as the authoritative source for self-guided
learning – with more than 50 million copies sold worldwide –
the **Teach Yourself** series includes over 500 titles in the fields of
languages, crafts, hobbies, business, computing and education.

British Library Cataloguing in Publication Data: a catalogue record
for this title is available from the British Library.

First published in UK 2010 by Hodder Education, part of
Hachette UK, 338 Euston Road, London NW1 3BH.

This edition published 2010.

The **Teach Yourself** name is a registered trade mark of
Hodder Headline.

Typeset by MPS Limited, a Macmillan Company.

Printed in Great Britain for Hodder Education, an Hachette UK
Company, 338 Euston Road, London NW1 3BH, by CPI Cox &
Wyman, Reading, Berkshire RG1 8EX.

The publisher has used its best endeavours to ensure that the URLs
for external websites referred to in this book are correct and active
at the time of going to press. However, the publisher and the
author have no responsibility for the websites and can make no
guarantee that a site will remain live or that the content will remain
relevant, decent or appropriate.

Hachette UK's policy is to use papers that are natural, renewable
and recyclable products and made from wood grown in sustainable
forests. The logging and manufacturing processes are expected to
conform to the environmental regulations of the country of origin.

Impression number   10 9 8 7 6 5 4 3 2
Year   2014

Acknowledgements

I would like to thank all those in my focus groups who provided feedback. A very special thank you to Victoria Roddam, my publisher at Hodder Education.

Note: To make the Sanskrit terms more accessible, no diacritics are used in the transliteration from the Sanskrit alphabet to the English alphabet.

Acknowledgements

Contents

Meet the author

Tantric sex has changed and enriched my life and, in writing this book, I'm sincerely hoping it will change and enrich yours, too.

After reading this book, you will go on to experience the greatest sex of your life. I guarantee it.

But Tantric sex is far more than a physical experience. It's using sex to create a euphoric, radically altered state of consciousness. A state of bliss. Not happiness. That's something different. *Bliss*. Bliss is hard to define but you certainly know it when you feel it. The early Tantrikas had bliss, or *ananda*, down to a fine art. They believed there were actually seven levels. The sixth level or *cidananda*, the bliss that comes from a sense of losing yourself in your partner, you will reach. In other words, you will achieve oneness.

The seventh level, *jagadananda*, very much depends on your own convictions. The early Tantrikas believed the radiance they experienced was just a foretaste of the ocean of bliss they would inhabit after death. They believed that in their rapture they could have some direct knowledge of the eternal, for 'Spirit can alone know Spirit'. In other words, an experience of *jagadananda* was an experience of *Brahman*, the originator of the universe.

Nowadays, there's enormous interest in the subject of Tantric sex. Numerous books have been written, thousands of courses have been run and all kinds of people claim to be doing it on a regular basis. But, in fact, in the vast majority of cases, it isn't Tantric sex at all. If you want to practise the authentic rituals, updated for the modern era, this book will tell you how.

I wish you *ananda*.
Paul Jenner, Spain, 2010

Only got a minute?

▶ Tantric sex is an experience of *ananda* (bliss).

▶ Tantric sex uses advanced physical and psychological techniques to rouse sexual energy.

▶ Tantrikas visualized sexual energy as a coiled serpent goddess, *Kundalini*, lying asleep at the base of the spine.

▶ In order to transform the sexual energy into bliss, Tantrikas visualized it passing up the spine through a succession of 'conversion points' or chakras.

▶ To prepare themselves for the new, blissful state of consciousness, Tantrikas would open their minds by breaking taboos.

▶ The Tantric gurus had understood that the universe is, in effect, a web of vibrations. That intuition can be exploited by the intoning of mantras.

- In order to prepare both their minds and their bodies, Tantrikas used a special kind of foreplay known as *nyasa*, visualizing the divine in each other. *Auparishtaka* (oral sex) is one such method of stimulation.

- The longer a *vira* (advanced male practitioner) withholds ejaculation, the more profound the altered blissful state of consciousness, and the more orgasms you can both enjoy.

- Non-ejaculation is a way of prolonging bliss, long after the Tantric sex session is over.

- When you both have good control of your sexual energies so you can always enjoy simultaneous orgasms.

- A *duti* (female practitioner) can learn to ejaculate.

- Tantrikas sometimes used *adhorata* (anal sex) as a quick route to *Kundalini* arousal.

- The most Tantric positions are those in which the woman is on top.

5 Only got five minutes?

1 Getting started with Tantric sex
  ▷ The difference between Tantric sex and 'normal' sex is that Tantric sex is both physical and spiritual.
  ▷ Tantric sex uses advanced physical and psychological techniques to rouse sexual energy and create an altered state of consciousness known as *ananda* (bliss).
2 *Kundalini*, the chakras and the subtle body
  ▷ Tantrikas believe there's a special source of energy at the base of the spine, envisaged as a serpent goddess called *Kundalini* (in the Hindu tradition) or *Candalini* (in the Buddhist tradition).
  ▷ After rousing *Kundalini*, Tantrikas meditate on a series of chakras as a way of transforming the sexual energy into bliss. Chakras can be seen as tools for visualization.
3 Breaking taboos
  ▷ Tantrikas believed a new blissful state of consciousness could only be achieved if they let go of their habitual ways of thinking. They used the technique of shock, breaking various taboos of their time.
  ▷ In Tantric sex you, too, will break one or more of your personal taboos.
4 Mantra – the Tantric vibrator
  ▷ One of the most impressive achievements of the Tantric gurus was the perception that the universe is effectively a web of vibrations.
  ▷ That intuition can be exploited by the intoning of mantras.
  ▷ Tantrikas today have the pleasure of being able to use modern technology – the vibrator.
5 Tantric foreplay and massage
  ▷ In order to prepare both their minds and their bodies Tantrikas used a special kind of foreplay known as *nyasa*.

- *Nyasa* involves taking turns to stimulate different parts of one another's bodies while visualizing the divine in each other.
- Modern science shows that skin-to-skin stimulation produces a chemical called oxytocin that increases sensual pleasure and the power of orgasms.

6 *Auparishtaka* – Tantric oral sex
- The early Tantrikas believed that sexual fluids had magical properties.
- *Auparishtaka* (oral sex) was therefore an important technique.
- Modern science has shown that women can absorb 'happy' chemicals from semen through the walls of their vaginas.

7 Ejaculation – how not to (for him), how to (for her)
- Men can learn to delay, or even completely withhold, ejaculation through breathing techniques and by gaining control of their muscles, and, most of all, their minds.
- Many women probably ejaculate without realizing it – learning to do it deliberately can take sex to a whole new level.

8 Multiple and simultaneous orgasms
- Men who have good control of ejaculation can experience multiple orgasms.
- Male multiple orgasms are not as powerful as ejaculatory orgasms in terms of physical contractions but they have a cumulative effect in the brain to produce exquisite 'mental orgasms'.
- When men prolong lovemaking to enjoy multiple orgasms, their partners will also have the time to experience multiple orgasms, and simultaneous orgasms become easy.

9 *Adhorata*
- Anal stimulation magnifies genital stimulation by, as the Tantrikas saw it, arousing *Kundalini* very directly – modern science shows that it involves the pudendal, vagus and femoral cutaneous nerves and possibly something called the coccygeal body.

▷ If you've not yet experienced *adhorata* (anal sex), try to keep an open mind – Tantra considers everything about the body to be holy, including the anal canal and rectum.

10 Tantric positions

▷ The majority of Tantric positions are those in which the woman is on top.

▷ With the woman on top and the man relatively still extended lovemaking becomes easy.

▷ A woman can use the 'secret language' – that is, stroke the man internally – once she's developed the muscles of her *yoni* (vagina).

11 The seven stages of bliss

▷ There are seven stages of bliss – the two highest are *cidananda* (a state of oneness with your partner) and *jagadananda* (a state of oneness with all of Creation).

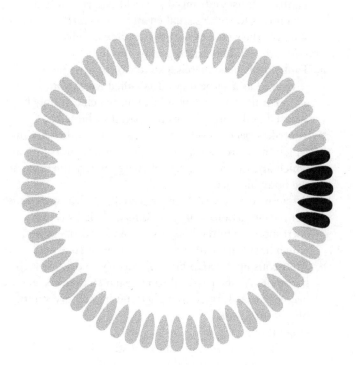

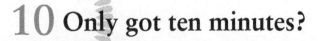

10 Only got ten minutes?

1 Getting started with Tantric sex
   ▷ The difference between Tantric sex and 'normal' sex is that Tantric sex is both physical and spiritual.
   ▷ Tantric sex uses advanced physical and psychological techniques to rouse sexual energy and create an altered state of consciousness known as *ananda* (bliss).

2 *Kundalini*, the chakras and the subtle body
   ▷ Tantrikas believe there's a source of sexual energy, envisaged as a serpent goddess called *Kundalini*, lying asleep at the base of the spine, and which can only be aroused and controlled using special techniques.
   ▷ Tantrikas believe everyone possesses a 'subtle body' in which there are *nadis,* or energy channels, and chakras, which are seen as vortexes of energy where the mind and the body interact.
   ▷ Western science has always rejected the idea of chakras, but recent advances suggest *nadis* and chakras may correspond with the body's system of neuropeptides, which have been called the 'molecules of emotion'.
   ▷ After rousing *Kundalini*, Tantrikas try to drive her up the spine. As she passes through each chakra, the energy becomes transformed to higher and higher levels until bliss is attained.

3 Breaking taboos
   ▷ Tantrikas believed a new blissful state of consciousness could only be achieved if they let go of their habitual ways of thinking. They used the technique of shock, breaking various taboos of their time.
   ▷ If you break some of your personal taboos and overcome your inhibitions you'll find it easier to reach the state of bliss known as *cidananda*, or oneness, with your partner.
   ▷ Being uninhibited doesn't mean doing things you don't want to do; it means doing things you do want to do but have been afraid of.

4 Mantra – the Tantric vibrator
   ▷ Modern science has shown that the whole universe and everyone in it vibrates in the 'cosmic dance', something the Tantric gurus intuited centuries ago.
   ▷ Tantrikas have long exploited that knowledge through the intoning of mantras – a mixture of vibration, breath and meaning.
   ▷ The moans and groans made during sex can be 'informal mantras' – be uninhibited and let them out.
   ▷ Buy a vibrator and experiment – the original Tantrikas would certainly have used them if they had been available.
   ▷ *Pranayama* (breath control) can be used to increase or decrease excitement.
5 Tantric foreplay and massage
   ▷ *Nyasa* is an ancient technique for arousing the body and influencing the mind.
   ▷ You arouse the body by taking turns to stimulate one another.
   ▷ You influence the mind by, at the same time, treating your partner as a goddess/god.
   ▷ If you treat your partner as a goddess/god he or she will become one.
   ▷ It's possible to 'train' less responsive parts of the body to become more sensitive over time, by 'yoking' them to more responsive parts.
   ▷ The importance of *nyasa* is underlined by the discovery that oxytocin, a chemical released by skin to skin contact, sensitizes the genitals and makes orgasms more powerful.
6 *Auparishtaka* – Tantric oral sex
   ▷ Originally, the whole point of Tantric sex was the production of sexual fluids, especially women's which were believed to confer gnosis (the intuitive understanding of spiritual truths) as well as *siddhis* (magical powers).
   ▷ *Auparishtaka* (oral sex) is a powerful technique, especially as the tongue is served by five pairs of cranial nerves.
   ▷ The best place to perform *auparishtaka* on a woman is the clitoris which has 8,000 nerve fibres, twice as many as in the penis.

- ▷ The best place to perform *auparishtaka* on a man is the underside of the glans of the penis.
- ▷ There's scientific evidence that a man's sexual fluids can be absorbed by a woman through the walls of her vagina, and that they promote happiness.

7 Ejaculation – how not to (for him), how to (for her)
- ▷ When a man intentionally keeps well away from the 'point of no return' (PNR), neither experiencing orgasm nor ejaculation, lengthy, meditative sex sessions become possible – with plenty of time to rouse *Kundalini* and no sexual hangover.
- ▷ During these long sessions a woman may also forego orgasm, or she may choose to enjoy orgasms by clitoral stimulation.
- ▷ All women can learn to ejaculate a burst of urine; it's not clear what proportion of women can also learn to ejaculate from the female prostate.
- ▷ The G-spot does exist. It's the rougher area of skin just inside the entrance to the vagina on the front wall. Female ejaculation is induced by stimulation of the G-spot with a pushing-out at the moment of orgasm.

8 Multiple and simultaneous orgasms
- ▷ Men can have multiple orgasms.
- ▷ Multiple orgasms in men can be with or without ejaculation, but only a small percentage of men can learn to experience them with ejaculation.
- ▷ Multiple male orgasms without ejaculation are 'brain orgasms' more than they're genital orgasms and lead directly to the state of bliss that is the aim of Tantric sex.
- ▷ Male multiple-type orgasms occur on the razor's edge of ejaculation.
- ▷ The first requirement for remaining on the razor's edge is an iron resolve, which can be helped by visualization and self-hypnosis. The principal physical technique is a series of violent exhalations with the tongue out and down.
- ▷ When men enjoy multiple orgasms, their partners also have the time to experience multiple orgasms.
- ▷ Women can learn to become multi-orgasmic through guilt-free, uninhibited masturbation.

▷ Simultaneous orgasms become simple once you're both multi-orgasmic.

9 *Adhorata*

▷ Anal stimulation magnifies genital stimulation – modern science shows that it involves the pudendal, vagus and femoral cutaneous nerves and possibly something called the coccygeal body.

▷ If you've not yet experienced *adhorata* (anal sex), try to keep an open mind – Tantra considers everything about the body to be holy, including the anal canal and rectum.

▷ Most men will enjoy being anally penetrated by their partner's fingers during sex – the prostate can be an additional source of pleasure.

▷ Employ plenty of foreplay to relax the sphincter and generous amounts of artificial lubricant – the anal canal and rectum produce none of their own.

10 Tantric positions

▷ Different positions offer different possibilities for breath control, the intoning of mantras, the meeting of eyes, energy circulation and altered states of consciousness, but the majority of Tantric positions are those in which the woman is on top.

▷ When the man is in control, however, he can more easily get very close to the PNR.

▷ The 'secret language' requires the woman to develop her muscles to the extent that she can stroke the *lingam* (penis) inside her *yoni* (vagina).

▷ In Tantric sex, whenever appropriate, men squat rather than kneel or lie.

11 The seven stages of bliss

▷ You'll be more likely to reach a state of bliss if you concentrate on the total experience, including wine, food, candles, incense, music and the right accessories.

▷ There are seven stages of bliss – the two highest *cidananda* (a state of oneness with your partner) and *jagadananda* (a state of oneness with all of Creation) are only likely to be reached after a lengthy session – as a guide, plan on three hours.

1

Getting started with Tantric sex

In this chapter you will learn:
- *what Tantric sex is*
- *the history of Tantric sex*
- *how to start enjoying Tantric sex right now.*

> *I follow the worship wherein there is enjoyment of wine,*
> *flesh and wife.*
>
> The Rudrayamala

Let's get down to some Tantric sex. Today. Right now, if you like.

All that's necessary is to start looking at sex in a new way. Stop thinking of it as a purely bodily experience and begin thinking of it as an experience of the *mind* as well.

What makes Tantric sex different is not its range of physical sexual techniques (potent though they are) but its range of *psychological* techniques and the *intention* behind the sex. The prolonged state of excitement which Tantric sex is capable of creating is only a beginning. Its aim is the attainment of a quite extraordinary state of mind known as *ananda* or bliss.

Ananda, in this context, is not the same as happiness. *Ananda* is something very special and, at its optimum, known as *jagadananda*, very rare. So rare, that most people never experience it in their lifetimes. But that's what we're going to be aiming for by the end of this book. So how will you know it? For one thing, however long it lasts (it could be minutes, it could be hours), and however you generate it, once you're *in* it, it's independent of external things. It's like lighting a flame that then burns on its own. Other names for it are *rasa* (juice-joy) and *maharaga* (the great emotion). It certainly *includes* happiness, it certainly *includes* a secure sense of being loved, but most important of all it is a sense of being *beyond* the kinds of fears and anxieties that are part of normal life.

You may have heard that Tantric sex is all about lengthy sex sessions during which the man does not ejaculate. That isn't strictly true. In fact, in early Tantric sex, ejaculation was considered vital, for reasons we'll see later. But it is true that the man must be able to *control* ejaculation and therefore *prolong* sex, so that *both* partners have the greatest chance of basking in this radiant state.

The techniques of Tantric sex require practice but there's no reason you shouldn't get a flavour of it immediately. And if neither of you is feeling especially turned on just now that's all to the good, because rushing to discharge sexual tension is the very opposite of Tantric sex. It's the action of a *pashu* (animal) rather than a *vira* (advanced male practitioner or 'hero') or a *duti* (female Tantrika). The key to success in Tantric sex is control. If that sounds rather cold and unromantic to you, reflect that pleasure in so many other passionate endeavours comes from the considered exercise of skill. The control needed to drive a high-performance sports car, ski down a mountain, ride a horse or play a musical instrument in no way detracts from the enjoyment. Rather, the reverse. And Tantric sex is no different.

Insight

Tantric sex is often described as a 'spiritual path'. In my opening remarks I deliberately avoided mentioning that because, although many people are seeking spiritual things, others are put off by that kind of talk. It certainly is *not* necessary to be religious to practise Tantric sex. **Tantra** probably grew up with Hinduism, and also became attached to Buddhism and *Jainism*, but there's no reason that suitable versions of Tantric sex shouldn't be practised by people of all religions or none. Christians can enjoy one style of Tantric sex. Atheists can enjoy a different style. But what about this 'spiritual path'? Is that really what Tantric sex is? And what does 'spiritual' mean, anyway? Let me tell you that if you're completely 'anti-spiritual' you can still follow all of the physical techniques of Tantric sex and have the greatest sex of your life. But it won't truly *be* Tantric sex because the word '*ananda*' doesn't just mean bliss, it means *spiritual* bliss. As to what that involves, we'll be finding out more as we go along. If talk of spiritual things makes you uncomfortable, then in your case, think of *ananda* as just a very beautiful kind of happiness.

A taste of Tantric sex

Here, then, is a shortcut to Tantric sex. It won't be the full experience. You'll have to read the whole book for that and practise the skills over the next few weeks. But it will give you a flavour of what people are talking about and convince you – if persuasion is needed – of the advantages of carrying on.

STEP 1 – PREPARE THE PLACE

The aim is to create a mood conducive to this new search for *ananda*. Light a few candles and sticks of incense. Put on some music. Make it something a little ethereal and mystical. The right music can act on the same parts of the brain that sex itself does, augmenting the effects. So choose carefully. Beside the bed, on a small table, place a glass of wine (if you drink alcohol) and something to feed one another with (for example, pistachio nuts). The early Tantrikas, as we'll see, had other ways of creating the right ambiance but for most modern couples this kind of approach works extremely well.

STEP 2 – PREPARE YOURSELVES

Be thinking about the sex you're going to have and how it will be unhurried, long and rapturous. Take a shower (together if you like) but then get dressed again – in your Tantric accoutrements, that is. Women who could afford it traditionally wore lots of jewellery – necklaces, bracelets, anklets and, most effective of all, some kind of chain around the waist, perhaps with a tassel hanging down between their thighs. Quite often they might also have worn a richly embroidered waistcoat or a tight-fitting *choli* – a modern crop-top looks about the same. Men, too, wore jewellery, if they were wealthy, and a waistcoat, or even a cloak, plus some kind of headgear. The idea was that sex was a very special occasion that partners should dress up for.

Shiva and Shakti

Tantrikas believed that during their sexualized rituals every male participant became a god (often called **Shiva** in the Hindu tradition) and every female participant became a goddess (often called **Shakti** in the Hindu tradition). That's why Tantrikas liked to dress up for lovemaking. Tantrikas believed that the whole universe was, in effect, created by Shiva and Shakti making love. So when you make love with your partner you are, symbolically, emulating the gods in the creation of the universe and should therefore adorn yourselves 'like gods'. On a purely physical level, the right accessories can be highly erotic. (For a better understanding of Tantric gods and goddesses see the factbox on p. 15.)

STEP 3 – PLAN ON A LONG SESSION

The techniques by which sex can be extended are fully explained in Chapters 7 and 8 and take some time to master. But for the moment we're going to have to resort to some 'trickery' to find a shortcut. Place a clock in a prominent, easily visible place where you're going to make love. Now, both of you decide for how long you're going to enjoy foreplay and intercourse. You should be aiming for significantly longer than you've ever managed before. Let's say a *minimum* of 20 minutes for foreplay, 20 minutes for intercourse and 20 minutes for cuddling afterwards. That's a pretty good way of spending an hour. But two hours, or three, would be even better.

The clock, I stress, is only a temporary device until you've mastered the mental and physical skills. Most men find it much easier to control ejaculation if they have a clear target to aim for. The notion of 'going on as long as possible' is simply too vague, but a target of, say, 20 minutes is something tangible.

Ananda

Alfred Kinsey, the pioneering American sex researcher (1894–1956) concluded that in his day, three-quarters of men ejaculated within two minutes of entering the vagina, which meant intercourse generally lasted two minutes. Nowadays, surveys suggest the norm is at least six minutes and possibly as much as ten. But even ten minutes is far from sufficient to create the kind of altered mental state that we're aiming for in Tantric sex.

Tantrikas believed the very special state of *ananda* they attained through sex was a foretaste of the permanent state of *ananda* into which they would eventually enter. In Tantra, **Brahma** (or **Brahman**), the Divine Consciousness, the origin of everything, literally *is ananda*. When you feel *ananda* you are having a direct experience of *Brahman*. But it can't be achieved by a 'quickie'. It requires a lengthy session to fully awaken the sexual energy known as **Kundalini**, and special techniques to drive her (for *Kundalini* is envisaged as a goddess) up the spine into the brain. (For more on *Kundalini* see Chapter 2.)

STEP 4 – FOREPLAY

Foreplay, or *nyasa*, is something very special and important in Tantric sex. It involves stimulating various parts of the body while affirming that your partner *is* the god Shiva or *is* the goddess Shakti. You can read a full explanation in Chapter 5 but, for now, just thinking of your partner as 'divine' certainly won't do your relationship or your sex life any harm.

A variant was the belief that during Tantric sex, women were inhabited by fierce and demanding female demigods known as *yoginis*. These *yoginis* very much enjoyed oral sex (*auparishtaka*) and the men who pleased them were believed to receive secret knowledge directly from the *yogini-vaktra* ('mouth of the *yogini*') – that's to say, the vulva (*yoni*). So, Shivas, (I'll often be referring to men as Shivas and women as Shaktis) get to work. If you want some ideas, turn to Chapter 6.

STEP 5 – ASANAS

The key to the special Tantric *asanas* (positions) is that the woman is generally on top. The goddess, as it were, actively 'takes' the man, who is relatively passive. The most famous Tantric position is *yab yum* (father mother) or the slightly easier version known as *sukhapadma asana* (easy lotus posture) where the man sits in the lotus, half-lotus or, simply, cross-legged, and the woman lowers her *yoni* (vulva/vagina) onto his *lingam* (penis) and sits on his lap with her legs wrapped around his waist. This reflects the active, non-submissive role of Shakti. It's also a position which creates relatively *little* stimulation. In Tantric sex, that's not a bad thing because it makes it easier to enjoy lengthy sessions. And it has other practical advantages, too. It's a convenient position for sharing food and wine. And, in an era when comfortable furniture was rare, it was a sensible solution to making love on the ground. However, if woman-on-top positions don't suit you, you might like to select some other positions from Chapter 10.

STEP 6 – MAITHUNA

Many women at first don't like the idea that they're not (as they see it) exciting their partners sufficiently for them to 'lose control'. So it's very important that when it comes to *maithuna* (intercourse) you're *both* intent on reaching the target. You, Shiva, need to keep going long enough for your partner to have at least one and, hopefully, several orgasms, while you yourself hover on the brink of ejaculation – at the end of the allotted time you can decide to ejaculate or not. Meanwhile, you, Shakti, should be doing your best to have plenty of orgasms while being careful not to over-stimulate your partner at critical moments.

So with the clock in easy view, *lingam* (penis) and *yoni* (vagina) are united. Whenever you, Shiva, get close to the 'point of no return', you cease all stimulation and let the excitement subside a little. Shakti must then also cease all stimulation. A very traditional Indian way of doing this is to share some wine and food that's been left within arm's reach. Alternatively, you could break apart for refreshments or simply to gaze at one another.

Each time you resume, you should aim to take the sensations to a new level. Tantrikas see this as driving *Kundalini* higher and higher up the spine until she enters the brain to bring about *samadhi* (enlightenment). The eventual aim is *moksha* (liberation from the cycle of death and rebirth). In your case you should focus on whatever your beliefs are. If your aim is a state of oneness with your partner, then meditate on that.

STEP 7 – EJACULATION?

To ejaculate or not to ejaculate? That is the question. In the earliest forms of Tantric sex the men always ejaculated. But, later, the whole emphasis changed towards an altered state of consciousness through non-ejaculation. If you, Shakti, are satisfied and if you, Shiva, can now withdraw without having ejaculated, then do so. Presumably that will be a new experience for you. Try it. You may feel a little frustrated but, on the plus side, you can have sex again very soon, and Shakti certainly won't be feeling neglected. But once you've mastered the techniques for **multiple orgasms** in Chapter 8, the frustration will go and you'll feel perfectly satisfied. In fact, more than that, you'll feel exhilarated and rather mystical.

Taoism

Tantric sex is often confused with the Chinese **Tao** or Dao (meaning 'Way') precisely because of non-ejaculation. The principal difference is the aim. Although Tao does not ignore spiritual issues, the whole point of Taoist sex is happiness, health and longevity *on Earth*. A man achieved that, the ancient Chinese believed, by balancing *yin* and *yang* (female and male) through intercourse *without ejaculation*. It was the squandering of semen, the Taoists believed, that led to illness and a premature death. You may have noted the focus on the *man's* longevity, but the woman's pleasure was extremely important in the Tao and the ancient Chinese texts devoted considerable space to that. A 'thousand loving thrusts' were considered necessary to satisfy a woman and, for maximum effect, they had to be delivered in various different patterns.

STEP 8 – AFTERGLOW

Now, spend 20 minutes revelling in the sensations you've created and just enjoying being naked together. Keep the music going and share something to eat and drink.

Why longer sex is better sex

According to an article in *The Sunday Times* in 2004, Sir Bob Geldof reportedly asked fellow pop star Sting, 'Why would you want it for eight hours? It must be so boring.' And then quipped: 'Thirty seconds, that's enough, that'll do me.'

In fact, a lot of people express the same sentiment. And that's quite strange. Nobody says that eating three meals a day is boring. Few people say that that lying on a Caribbean beach several hours a day for a fortnight is boring. Or skiing every day of a two-week holiday is boring. And yet many people are startled by the idea of, say, a whole evening of sex. That's possibly because the Western style of sex is so often simply about discharging 'unpleasant' sexual tension, of gaining relief, and doing it as quickly as possible.

The Tantrika sees things very differently. The *vira* cultivates lust, cultivates sexual tension, enjoys it, doesn't wish to discharge it. On the contrary, the *vira* wants to build it up and use it. The *vira*, as we've seen, employs it to create a blissfully altered state of consciousness. But even if you, Shiva, have no interest in spiritual matters there are several reasons why the same approach is still good for you. And as for you, Shakti, your natural multi-orgasmic capacity will know no constraints.

Let's stick with the analogy of a meal. If you wanted to create a truly great menu, you would think in terms of several courses. You might have pauses between. Little dishes to clean the palate and sharpen the appetite – an aperitif, perhaps, some sauces, a sorbet and so on. You would expect the meal to last a good while. And you wouldn't rely solely on the food. There would be interesting and amusing conversation, music, and, finally, something to create that lasting glow – a brandy, perhaps.

So it is with Tantric sex.

So what actually is Tantric sex?

Tantric sex is just one aspect of a whole body of beliefs and practices known as Tantra. Because Tantra was not founded by any single person and has never had any sort of ruling body to define its beliefs, so its teachings have varied from century to century, place to place, and **guru** to guru.

There's not even agreement about the dictionary definition of the word 'Tantra' itself. Its first known use in a text goes back to at least the fifth century BCE when it was used to mean an interweaving of rites. Some scholars point to '*tan*' as a Sanskrit root signifying something to do with weaving so that Tantra becomes a belief in the interwovenness of all things. However, given that medieval Indian texts on all kinds of subjects were also known as Tantras, I opt for the more prosaic interpretation that a Tantra was simply a book of instructions or rules, including but not confined to mystical teachings. When the British arrived in India they mistakenly started talking about Tantra and Tantrikas in the same way that the mythical visitor from Mars might call certain people 'Biblers'.

Just to complicate things, the 'cult of ecstasy', that Tantra is often said to be, mostly refers to a sect within Tantra known as the *Kaula*. It would be more accurate, then, to talk of '*Kaula* sex' than 'Tantric sex'. But, probably, no *sadhaka* (male follower of the rituals) or *sadhika* (female follower) would ever have used either term. And, unfortunately, Tantric sex has been hijacked in the last few years by self-proclaimed gurus who seem to know little about the authentic rites. Nevertheless, I'm also using the phrase 'Tantric sex' because it's something that everybody has come to recognize.

No one even knows when Tantra (to continue the mistake) began as a spiritual path. The earliest surviving documents to be given the title 'Tantra' date from the seventh century, and are Buddhist, but most scholars believe Tantra arose out of Hinduism. Certainly the origins of Tantra go back much, much further.

Many Hindus today refer to 'Tantra-mantra' in the same way that we might say 'mumbo-jumbo'. But we shouldn't be surprised that so much in Tantra looks ridiculous from a modern perspective. Those early Tantric 'scientists' were struggling with many of the same questions that we still struggle with today, yet without any of our scientific instruments. Some of their conclusions were, indeed, 'black magic' of a kind quite laughable now. What's astonishing, however, is how many correct or, at least, plausible answers they came up with.

Tantrikas, like Hindus, have always believed in what we now call the Big Bang theory. That's to say, they believe the universe was once the size of a dot and will return to a dot. And that the process will be repeated over and over. Endlessly. The expansion is powered by the ONE, the Divine Consciousness, or *Brahman*. *Brahman* was lonely and split into two, creating a god often called Shiva, and a goddess often called Shakti. It was their lovemaking that created the visible universe, sending out patterns of vibrations that coalesced into the forms that we, tricked by *maya* (the covering that conceals true reality) perceive as solid. So that is very much in line with modern quantum theory.

When Shiva and Shakti stop making love, so the vibrations will cease and the universe will return to a dot. When Tantrikas make love they, as it were, become Shiva and Shakti, helping create the vibrations that maintain the cosmos. So keep on playing your part as often as possible.

The Tantric texts

Only a few of the many Tantric texts have so far been translated into English. One of the earliest and most important is Chapter 29 of the tenth century *Tantraloka* by the sage **Abhinavagupta**, to which a commentary was added in the thirteenth century by a guru called **Jayaratha**. It's the chapter that deals with the sexualized ritual known as the *rahasyacarya* (secret ceremony) or *cakrapuja* (circle worship) but in terms so obscure that it's mainly of interest to scholars. Nevertheless, keep the names in mind because they were key players in the development of Tantra.

The *Mahanirvana Tantra* is more easily understood but, having been written in the nineteenth century under British rule, presents a rather tamer picture of Tantric belief and practice. It was translated by a man who used the pseudonym Arthur Avalon. It's perhaps not surprising if

(Contd)

he preferred to play down the sexual aspects of Tantra because his real name was Sir John Woodroffe, who became Advocate General of Bengal and, in 1915, Chief Justice of the High Court of India at Calcutta.

For more on Tantric texts and books on Tantra see Taking it further on p. 263.

Women and Tantric sex

Some scholars have argued that Tantra is a cult of 'goddess worship' and that, therefore, for at least a part of its history, women were in charge, enjoying their orgasms and ejaculations (see Chapter 7) by 'using' men. For modern women it can be that way but, historically, nothing could have been further from the truth. An archaeologist of the future, unearthing today's magazines and websites, with images of women displaying their bodies to be 'worshipped', might also jump to the conclusion that women were in charge at the start of the third millennium. But, as we know, that would not be accurate.

The harsh truth is that in authentic Tantric sex, it was men who used women as a means of gaining spiritual enlightenment and, as they believed, magical powers. Although there were female gurus, just as there are female politicians today, and although certain secret practices were probably passed on by women, it was very much a man's world.

For an insight into the position of women in the India of two and a half thousand years ago, we can turn to the *Brihadaranyaka Upanishad*. It instructs the man to open the woman's thighs, repeating the **mantra**: 'Spread yourselves apart, Heaven and Earth.' He should then insert his member, join mouth to mouth, and stroke her 'three times from head to foot'. So this is sounding like an early form of Tantra. But what if the woman 'does not willingly yield her body'? In that case he should try to 'buy her with presents'. If she is still 'unyielding' he should then 'strike her with a stick or with his hand and overcome her...' That certainly doesn't sound very much like women being in charge.

The Tantras themselves paint a similar picture of male domination. The *Brihad Nila Tantra* instructs the man, 'Have there a young and beautiful girl...' The *Yoni Tantra* says, 'The devotee should place a Shakti in a circle...' Jayaratha's commentary to the *Tantraloka* says the person who wishes to perform ritualized sex should 'bring a sexual partner, but not if *he* is deluded by desire' (my italics). Later Jayaratha says, '*He* should enjoy beautiful women...'

You might object that these are carefully selected quotes (which they're not). But what's most significant is not what some Tantras say but what no Tantras ever say. You'll search in vain for an instruction such as, '*She* should bring a man,' or '*She* should enjoy a handsome man.' Everything is written from the male point of view, nothing from the woman's.

Compared with the position of women *generally*, however, it's certainly possible that Tantra was a little less unequal. After all, just as the man became an incarnation of a god (usually Shiva in the Hindu tradition) so the woman became an incarnation of a goddess (usually Shakti, or **Kali** in the Hindu tradition). What's more, Tantra recognized that all women contained male elements and that all men contained female elements.

So should you, if you're a woman, reject Tantric sex? You should certainly reject the Tantric sex of a millennium ago. But in this book I'm extracting the elements that are good for modern relationships and modern sex, and for women just as much as men.

Insight

Women I've interviewed who practise Tantric sex speak of enjoying the extensive and varied foreplay. They relish being

(Contd)

able to have as many orgasms as they wish. They find their partners more attentive and appreciative at all times. They have deeper and more meaningful communication, and they treasure the moments of oneness.

Tantric sex and love

Tantric sex is, self-evidently, about using *sex*, not love, as a means to an end. Just as two people can have sex without being in love, so they can have Tantric sex without being in love. Indeed, in so-called 'left-hand' Tantra, men and women had sex indiscriminately. The belief was that every man was Shiva and every woman was Shakti and it didn't make any difference who you had sex with. I have interviewed Tantrikas today who tell me the more strangers you have sex with 'the higher you go'.

However, I don't share that belief. In this book I follow the 'right-hand path', which some nowadays call 'white Tantra' because, in my opinion, the greatest rapture will be reached together with a partner you love. There's every reason to follow Tantric sex practices as best you can right from your first encounter with a new partner. But I don't think you'll ever reach the ultimate state of ecstasy with someone you're not in love with. That's not a moral judgement. For a start, achieving rapture requires a degree of complicity that two strangers are unlikely to achieve. Secondly, although you may well enjoy sex on a purely physical level with someone you hardly know, you won't attain very much on the emotional and spiritual planes. Thirdly, you probably won't be very uninhibited with someone you don't love; you may resort to alcohol to overcome those inhibitions, but a large quantity of alcohol will make ecstasy impossible. Fourth, the 'meeting of eyes' is an important phase in my kind of Tantric sex, as is the co-ordination of breathing. Will you really stare for several minutes into the eyes of someone you don't love? And, even if you do, will that help create the same state of rapture as if you loved that person?

If you are a single, unattached man or woman, you have every reason to learn the secrets of Tantric sex. It will still be the best sex you ever had. But it won't be the ultimate sexual experience until you find a partner you love – a partner you are utterly willing to dissolve your own consciousness into.

CAN I BE A TANTRIKA IF MY PARTNER ISN'T?

The *Mahakala Samhita* is quite clear that *sadhaka* and *sadhika* must be at the same level of Tantric knowledge and skill. 'In this way only,' it says, 'is success attained and not otherwise even in ten million years.'

Nevertheless, I take the view that one Tantrika is better than no Tantrika. I'd be astonished if, after you've started exploring the Tantric path, your partner doesn't follow. It's just too good.

Gods and goddesses in Tantra

Westerners are often confused by the large number of 'gods' that exist in Tantra. But this is really a problem of translation from the Sanskrit. A better translation might be 'saints' as understood by the Roman Catholic Church. Just as Catholics may pray not only to God but also to individual saints who, it is thought, might be especially sympathetic, so Tantrikas might try to invoke a particular deity. In fact, every village would have had its own particular god or saint, in addition to the ones worshipped everywhere, so that the actual number was enormous. These Tantric gods, like the Catholic saints, were originally human but were elevated to semi-divine status.

Scholars now believe that many of them were, in fact, the leaders of the Aryans, who invaded India from around 1500 BCE. The three-millennia old *Rig Veda*, which introduced various gods, is not, according to this view,

(Contd)

an account of the struggle between Good (the *devas*) and Evil (the *dasas*), but between the Aryans on the one hand and the earlier inhabitants of India (the Asuras, Raksas, Gandharvas and so on). The defeated became the lower members of India's caste system.

I'm going to stick with the accepted translation, 'gods'. But remember that we're not talking about God in the, say, Christian or Muslim sense; we're talking about something similar to semi-divine saints in the Catholic sense.

Insight

Of course, you may not believe in semi-divine beings. I don't, personally. But that doesn't stop me from practising Tantric sex. I enjoy this aspect of Tantra as a sort of colourful folklore that, in the era before modern technology, provided people with an explanation of the phenomena they experienced. As we'll be seeing, behind many of the beliefs and practices in Tantric sex, there's amazingly good science.

10 THINGS TO REMEMBER

1 *Tantric sex is an experience of* ananda *(spiritual bliss).*

2 Ananda *is not the same as happiness;* ananda *is like a flame that, once lit, burns on its own.*

3 *Tantric sex is often described as a 'spiritual path' and, indeed, 'bliss' does include a spiritual element. If you don't wish to follow a spiritual path you can still use all the advanced physical techniques for the greatest sex of your life, but it won't truly be Tantric sex.*

4 *Tantrikas believed they were gods and goddesses, or were inhabited by gods and goddesses when they made love, so you should prepare and adorn your bodies accordingly.*

5 *It takes time to drive* Kundalini *(sexual energy) into the brain to achieve the altered state of consciousness that's essential to Tantric sex, so a session should never be less than an hour, and preferably much longer.*

6 Nyasa *(foreplay) and* auparishtaka *(oral sex) are both very important.*

7 *A* vira *(advanced male practitioner) doesn't always withhold ejaculation but must be capable of controlling ejaculation.*

8 *Control over ejaculation makes it possible for* both *a* vira *and a* duti *(female practitioner) to experience multiple orgasms.*

9 *Although there were some female gurus, Tantric sex was originally all about men using women to gain spiritual enlightenment and magical powers; for this book I've extracted what's suitable for modern couples, and with as much emphasis on women's pleasure as on men's.*

10 *You don't have to be in love to practise Tantric sex but it will be much more powerful if you are.*

HOW TANTRIC ARE YOU NOW?

Here's a little quiz to see how Tantric you are. Tick the statements you agree with now. Then see how many you tick after you've finished reading the book and practised Tantric sex for a while.

☐ I often feel a deep sense of connection with my partner.
☐ I often feel a deep sense of connection with the people around me.
☐ I often feel a deep sense of connection with all life.
☐ I believe that sex is central to a relationship because it's then I become one with my partner and no longer feel alone.
☐ My body is a tool of my mind and I'm not inhibited about using it in sex.
☐ It's important to be open to new ideas.
☐ When I'm making love with my partner I feel energy rising up my spine into my brain.
☐ When I'm making love with my partner I often feel that we're one person.
☐ When I'm making love with my partner I'm not consciously aware of anything else at all.
☐ Nothing creates such a state of ecstasy as sex.
☐ I sometimes have the feeling that nothing in normal life matters because we're really all part of something much, much bigger than we realize.
☐ I believe that sex can create an altered state of consciousness that allows us to perceive the reality of the universe more clearly.
☐ I feel a warm glow that lasts for hours after sex.
☐ I feel quite mystical for hours after having sex.
☐ I feel desire for my partner all the time and it's a nice feeling.

2

....

Kundalini, the chakras and the subtle body

In this chapter you will learn:

- *how to direct energy within your own body*
- *how to exchange energy with your partner*
- *how to rouse* Kundalini, *the ultimate sexual energy*
- *how to use chakras to transform sexual energy into spiritual bliss.*

> *The Kundalini...unites Herself. The nectar which flows from such union floods the human body. It is then that the* sadhaka, *forgetful of all in this world, is immersed in ineffable bliss.*
>
> Arthur Avalon (Sir John Woodroffe), Introduction to the *Mahanirvana Tantra*

Now let's expand on some of the ideas I introduced in Chapter 1. Both of you take off your shoes and socks/tights and anything else you feel like. At least have *some* naked skin. Lie down together somewhere comfortable and have a nice cuddle. Work up a bit of a tingle.

Okay, here comes the special part. Once you've created a little excitement, let your feet touch your partner's. Something about it should feel *strange* in a pleasant sort of way. It's not an overwhelming sensation. In fact, it's quite subtle. Yet something about it seems *right*. If you take your feet away there's a sense of loss and when you put them back a kind of harmony is restored.

So what's going on? Well, Tantrikas believe it's all to do with the circulation of energy, and sexual energy in particular.

_____

Energy

You may already be very comfortable with the idea of creating energy, moving it around your body and even transferring it to other people (or receiving it from them). Or you may be highly sceptical. If you are, that's fine. Being open to new ideas doesn't mean accepting everything and anything without subjecting it to proper scrutiny. But as sexual energy is pretty fundamental to Tantric sex I'm going to spend a little time trying to convince you – or, rather, getting you to convince yourself – that it *is* possible to move energy in the way I've described.

Have a go
In this little experiment you're going to send energy into your hands in the form of heat, via increased blood flow – a useful trick when you want to massage your partner. There's a fairly simple principle at work. When you're tense, blood flow to your internal organs increases at the expense of your extremities (in readiness for 'fight or flight'). So you first need to relax and then you need to concentrate on blood flow.

- ▶ **Step 1:** *Ideally you should have a probe you can attach to your finger to measure the temperature but, in the absence of one, touch your hand against some warmer part of your body or a friend's body to make a comparison.*
- ▶ **Step 2:** *Relax for two or three minutes by breathing in through your nose to the count of seven, and out through your nose to the count of eleven. Continue this rhythm of shorter inhalations and longer exhalations throughout Steps 3–5.*
- ▶ **Step 3:** *Visualize sitting on a warm beach with the sun blazing down. You place your palms on the sand and it's hot.*
- ▶ **Step 4:** *Imagine that your hands are hollow and filling with warm blood which, as your hands rest on the sand, is heated still further. Really 'see' your hands and feel the heat.*

▶ **Step 5:** *Tell yourself how relaxed you feel, how you can sense the blood coursing into your hands, and how they feel hot and heavy with the blood.*

▶ **Step 6:** *After ten minutes, again touch your hand against the reference point; it should be noticeably warmer.*

Different kinds of technique are used in the above exercise. If you find one of them works better than another for you then stick with that.

SEXUAL ENERGY

Being able to increase the blood flow to your hands is one thing, but what about, say, to your genitals? That's rather more useful for sex. Try using a variation of the above technique, first getting relaxed all over and then getting especially relaxed between your legs. As for moving sexual energy from one part of your body to another, the key is this Tantric saying:

Where the mind goes the energy follows.

Have a go
All you have to do is focus for a time on part of the body and the energy will 'go' there. For example, you probably weren't aware of your left ear until you read this. Now you are. And if you continue to focus on your left ear you will, after a few moments, become aware of the blood pumping through it.

▶ **Step 1:** *Begin to arouse yourself in the usual way.*

▶ **Step 2:** *As your arousal increases, ask yourself: 'Where is my focus?' Of course, it's on your clitoris or penis. Now see what happens if you quite deliberately move your attention to another part of your body, say your left foot, while continuing self-stimulation. Almost certainly you'll find the excitement in your genitals waning.*

▶ **Step 3:** *Now, rather than just focusing attention, go a stage further by visualizing the response of the body part. For example, 'see' your nipples becoming larger. They probably will.*

▶ **Step 4:** *Play around with this for a while until you feel ready to try it out with your partner. When you change focus, it should be as if you've thrown a switch. Suddenly your genitals just aren't as responsive as they were. Some of the excitement has gone. Some of the 'energy' has moved from your clitoris/ penis to your foot, nipple or wherever.*

EXCHANGING SEXUAL ENERGY WITH SOMEONE ELSE

So it's fairly clear that you can consciously move energy around your own body. And, obviously, you can exchange heat energy with someone else. But can you do more?

Have a go
▶ **Step 1:** *The first thing is to generate some sexual energy. Begin sex however you like, then get into the* yab yum *position (Shakti on Shiva's lap, facing him – see Chapter 10), the* lingam *firmly inserted into the* yoni.
▶ **Step 2:** *Synchronize your breathing. With your heads close together you should be able to hear one another. (But if you can't naturally maintain the same breathing rhythm then don't struggle with this because it will detract from what follows.)*
▶ **Step 3:** *Focus on your united genitals. Don't just imagine your own. Visualize the energy being created by them together.*
▶ **Step 4:** *Now visualize the energy moving. One of you will have to act as 'god of energy' and announce where the focus is to be. Remember you're trying to circulate the energy through* both *of you. So you might say: 'Next visualize the energy at the base of* my *spine…now visualize the energy moving up* my *spine…now it's in the top of* my *head…now it's in my tongue passing to your tongue…now it's moving down* your *chest…' The usual pattern of movement is from the united genitals up the first person's spine into the head, via the tongues into the other person's head, down his or her chest to the united genitals once more, up the second person's spine, and so on, round and round. Don't rush. Make sure you both have time to settle on each new focus and feel it as much as possible before moving to the next. Give the body time to react.*

- ▶ **Step 5:** *After a few circuits, swap roles, so the other partner becomes the 'god of energy'. Does that make any difference? Discuss to what extent you could feel your own energy in your own body, your partner's energy in your body, and your energy in your partner's body.*
- ▶ **Step 6:** *Now, instead of following a regular, predictable sort of circuit through your combined bodies, try taking turns to call out body parts at random. So it might go like this. 'Your clitoris.' 'My right nipple.' 'Your right forefinger.' 'Your left nipple' 'My glans.' And so on. Again, be sure to allow enough time for each of you to refocus and for the body to respond. When you've tried that for a while, discuss whether or not this random movement of energy is more or less effective than the 'circulation of energy' exercise.*

KUNDALINI – *THE SERPENT GODDESS*

Tantrikas don't settle for the body's standard energy output, which is what we've been doing up till now. The whole aim of Tantric sex is to unleash a 'supercharge' to create a state of rapture far beyond anything in normal experience. Hindu Tantrikas call this energy *Kundalini*, while Buddhist Tantrikas (who have a slightly different view) call it *Candali* or *Candalini*. According to the sixteenth century *Sat-Cakra-Nirupana* (The Description of the Six Chakras) by Purnananda-Svami:

> *She [Kundalini] is the world-bewilderer... Like the spiral of the conch-shell, Her shining snake-like form goes three and a half times round Siva, and Her lustre is as that of a strong flash of lightning. Her sweet murmur is like the indistinct hum of swarms of love-mad bees. She produces melodious poetry... It is She who maintains all the beings of the world by means of inspiration and expiration and shines in the cavity of the root Lotus like a chain of brilliant lights.*

(Translated by Sir John Woodroffe, 1919)

So *Kundalini* is a divine female serpent who, according to Tantric belief, remains coiled asleep at the base of the spine in the

Muladhara chakra (see **chakras** factbox on p. 31) until awoken by certain special practices, of which Tantric sex is one. She is the 'inner Shakti', the creative power in both men and women, who seeks union with the 'inner Shiva', who lives in the head. (Interestingly, in the West, too, creativity is often seen as linked with the sex drive.) The aim of Tantric sex is to facilitate her wish, first arousing her then helping her up the spine and into the brain so the 'cosmic couple' can be together. In the process, enormous energy is released – far surpassing that of 'ordinary' sex – which can, as it were, smash through the crown of the head into the 'ultimate reality' causing a bliss-creating nectar or *rasa*-juice to flood the body.

Colourful rubbish? Yes and no. As you'll discover, things in Tantric sex can be taken literally, as many did, or they can be understood on the level of symbol and allegory. Let's take a look at how energy is actually generated in the human body. It may not have anything to do with snakes, but it is to do with something just as amazing…bugs.

The astonishing fact is that in every one of the cells of our bodies there are tiny components called mitochondria, little factories that produce most of our energy in the form of electricity. Billions of years ago, so it's believed, the ancestors of those mitochondria were free-living bacteria. At some point they invaded, or were swallowed up by, the kinds of cell that now constitute human beings, to live symbiotically together. And in every cell there are not just one or two, but thousands of them.

So, electricity is one of the energy sources that powers the body. Everything is harmoniously composed of roughly equal numbers of protons (which carry a positive charge) and electrons (which carry a negative charge) otherwise the energy would blow them up. When you touch anything, you are actually feeling the electrons. So it's not difficult to imagine that an electric charge could pass from one person to another. The problem is that no one so far has been able to measure it.

One explanation might be that the voltages are so tiny. But, in that case, could there really be a significant effect anyway? Well, yes there could. Although the body runs on only about 0.1 to 0.2 volts, that works out at several million volts per metre given that the membranes separating the circuits are five nanometres (one millionth of the thickness of a fingernail). Relatively speaking, that's a higher voltage than is found in a thunderstorm. It's not implausible that a so far undetectable current could have an effect. And, in fact, researchers have discovered a clue. They found that when one person tried to send energy to another, the sender's electrocardiogram (ECG) signal registered on the receiver's electroencephalogram (EEG). The effect was greatest when the receiver's right hand was held in the sender's right or left, and weakest when left hands were joined. But there was even a measurable effect when two people sat close together without actually touching. It's not hard to imagine that, during sex, the current (or whatever it turns out to be) would be much greater.

Electrical energy is not the whole story. There's also chemical energy to consider. Tantric sex is capable of creating massive, long-lasting chemical changes in the brain. In particular, these techniques alter levels of dopamine and PEA which, in tandem, produce a blissful high, as well as oxytocin, which creates a powerful sense of affection and attachment, and serotonin, which is involved in mystical feelings. I'll have a lot more to say about mind-altering chemicals in Chapter 8.

Knowing all this to be the truth, the early Tantric view perhaps doesn't seem so ridiculous after all. It's not difficult to imagine the Tantrikas, living in an era before modern science, trying to work out what was going on, and explaining it to themselves in this colourful image of *Kundalini*. After all, they had no knowledge of electricity or neurotransmitters, and sexual energy *does* seem to rise up from the genitals, and it *does* seem to enter the brain, and it *does* seem as if that energy can be transferred from one partner to the other, and there *does* seem to be a point reached at which, with your brain almost literally exploding, you seem to be on the verge of solving the mysteries of the universe. If it helps to visualize this rising energy as a serpent goddess then why not?

And there's more. Western science *has* discovered something strange – approximately in the area of the body where *Kundalini* is said to 'sleep' – something the Tantrikas are calling the '***Kundalini* gland**'.

The *Kundalini* gland

For a long time, *Kundalini* seemed to be nothing more than a picturesque way of explaining the power of sex. Then, in 1860, came the discovery of Luschka's body, also known as the coccygeal body, a long thin object between the rectum and the base of the spine.

Back then it wasn't possible to discover anything about the function of Luschka's body, but knowledge was advanced slightly by a light and electron microscope study in 1998 (Sargon, Hamdi Celik, Demiryürek and Dagdeviren) which described it as 'several blood vessels encapsulated by a connective tissue capsule' and noted that the small arteries within had an unusual lining. Then in 2000, a group of scientists working on mice published research in *Neuroendcrinology Letters* saying that the coccygeal body had a possible role in the creation of various blood cells and that it also had the ability to modulate the sympathetic nervous system, acting on noradrenaline (norepinephrine), adrenaline and dopamine. These are key chemicals in the sexual experience.

Given its position, the most direct way of stimulating the *Kundalini* gland is via the rectum, and any man or woman who has experienced good anal sex will know that it increases and extends the level of arousal significantly. But is the coccygeal body genuinely the source of *Kundalini* or are the well-known vagus and pudendal nerves the real source of the mind-altering excitement? That's a subject we'll be looking at in detail in Chapter 9, although until the scientists take things further, we can't know the answer for sure. But, as non-scientists, there is one thing we can do. That is explore Tantric sexual methods to see for ourselves if some extra special source of sexual energy is unleashed.

Have a go
All of this book is, in effect, about stimulating *Kundalini*, and you won't be able to do it properly until you've read the whole of it and practised for a while. So although this chapter is about rousing and directing *Kundalini* you're not actually going to be able to achieve the ultimate effect until you've prepared your body and your mind. For your body, here are some **PC muscle** exercises to get started on (PC stands for the **pubococcygeus muscle** but in popular use has come to mean all the muscles of the pelvic floor). If you're not yet aware of your PC, try halting the flow next time you urinate – *that's* the PC muscle. (If you can't halt it, your PC muscle is definitely too weak.)

▶ **Exercise 1:** *Contract and release your PC muscle as many times as possible in ten seconds. Repeat three times with breaks of ten seconds in between. As you get better, increase the number of contractions per session and the number of sessions per day.*

▶ **Exercise 2:** *Slowly contract and then hold your PC muscle for five seconds. Repeat ten times initially, building up to fifty times a day.*

▶ **Exercise 3:** *After warming up with short contractions, slowly squeeze and hold your PC muscle as tightly as possible for thirty seconds. Rest and repeat five times. Over a few weeks aim to build up the period for which you can hold your PC muscle to as much as two minutes.*

▶ **Exercise 4:** *Instead of steadily increasing and releasing the contraction as in the previous exercise, do it in five steps, holding for five seconds at each intermediate stage and for thirty seconds at maximum contraction.*

THE CHAKRAS AND ANANDA

One day 'a bearded yogi dressed in white and wearing a turban' showed up at the office of Candace Pert Ph.D., the scientist who discovered the opiate receptor in the human brain. According to her own account in her book *Molecules Of Emotion* (1999), the yogi wanted to know 'if endorphins [the body's own opiate-like pleasure chemicals] were concentrated along the spine in a way that corresponded to the Hindu chakras'. At that time Pert says she had no idea what the yogi was on about but, trying to be helpful, she pulled out a diagram of the two chains of nerve bundles running along either side of the spinal cord. Comparing it with the yogi's diagram of the chakras, Pert for the first time 'seriously considered that there might be a connection between my work and the Eastern viewpoint'.

And what was the yogi on about? Pert doesn't say exactly what his diagram showed but it probably would have depicted five, six or seven special places between the base of the spine and the crown of the head. If you had a difficulty with the concept of *Kundalini* you're going to have even more of a problem with chakras, because in Tantric belief, chakras transform sexual energy into *ananda*, which, as you now know, is the whole aim of Tantric sex. (I'll be making the point again and again that if you follow the physical practices of Tantric sex you'll have the greatest sex of your life, but it won't actually be genuine Tantric sex unless you include *ananda*.)

The origin of the chakra concept, as far as we know it, was not very scientific. The earliest accounts, in the eighth century Buddhist *Caryagiti* and *Hevajra Tantras*, said there were only four chakras and, on the basis that the human body was a microcosm of the universe, identified them with four geographical locations which seem to have been Gauhati in Assam, Jalandhara in upper Punjab, a place called Purnagiri which was also possibly in Punjab, and the Swat Valley. Later the chakras seem to have become circles of divine maidens, dressed in different colours, and who could grant *siddhis* (magical powers).

So this looks like mere superstition, especially when you know that the different religions that adopted the chakra concept don't all agree on numbers. Buddhists have stuck with four principal chakras, for example, whilst some Tantrikas talk of five and some of seven, plus various 'minor' chakras (see chakras factbox, p. 31). Some gurus even say the number can be infinite. Which, on the face of it, is all very confusing. If doctors couldn't agree how many, say, kidneys there were in the body, no one would take the kidney very seriously. So should we take chakras seriously?

The technique of the early yogic scientists, from whom the Tantrikas drew a great deal, was to experiment on themselves. As we know, they accomplished astonishing feats such as being able to slow their hearts and hold their breath for several minutes. So it would have been a very obvious to them that certain emotions were felt in specific parts of the body. For example, we've all felt sexual desire in the groin and love at the heart. Given that sexual desire seems to rise up and may be followed by love, it wasn't illogical to imagine that there might be some mechanism at the heart for transforming the one into the other. It's these places where transformations take place that are known as chakras, meaning 'circles' (also spelt *cakras*), possibly because feelings do seem to go round and round. They're also known as *padmas* (lotus flowers) because, in the right conditions, they can 'open' and 'bloom'.

Western science's first reaction to chakras was that they were simply a primitive explanation of physical organs:

Muladhara chakra	Testes/ovaries
Swadhisthana chakra	Adrenal glands
Manipura chakra	Pancreas and liver
Anahata chakra	Thymus gland
Vishuddha chakra	Thyroid gland
Ajna chakra	Pituitary gland
Sahasrara chakra	Pineal gland

This seemed logical enough, but in *The Serpent Power* (1919), Sir John Woodroffe, the leading British authority of his day, wrote that 'it is a mistake, in my opinion, to identify the Cakras [chakras] with the physical plexuses... These latter are things of the gross body, whereas the Cakras are extremely subtle vital centres of various Tattvik operations.'

In other words, chakras do not exist as physical organs that can be seen. In Tantra, the physical body, known as *Sthula-sarira*, is the outer sheath for a '**subtle body**', known as *Suksma-sarira*, which can't be seen. The crown of the head is the meeting point between the everyday and the transcendent and, there, an invisible opening lets in vital energy (*prana*) which spreads through the body via a network of channels or *nadis*. The principal *nadi* runs along the spine and is called ***susumna*** (some gurus say it's inside the spine, some outside).

It's a part of this belief system that the world we sense through our eyes, ears, and so on, is nothing but a projection. In other words, it's not a question of light coming from real objects but of people projecting images *from* their eyes. The 'screen' onto which they project is called the *root-prakriti*. The *sadhaka* must learn to cease projecting these images and, instead, to concentrate the energy and send it through the system of *nadis* to the point of the crown where it will blow a hole right through into the ultimate reality.

At first sight this is yet more pre-scientific Eastern mumbo-jumbo and can never be reconciled with Western science. The yogi who visited Candace Pert wanted to know if she could find any common ground. Quite possibly she has done.

Cells have receptors all over their surfaces, often explained as being like keyholes. The 'keys' are known as ligands and are divided into three chemical types, the neurotransmitters, the steroids and – Pert's special interest – the peptides. The cell's behaviour is determined by which ligands are in their respective keyholes at any moment. The ligands – and this is the essential point – simply drift by in the stream of fluid that surrounds every cell. There's no 'ligand tube'. Nothing resembling an artery or a nerve. The whole ligand-receptor system is, in effect, invisible and yet, as Pert describes it, it's a 'second nervous system'.

Here's the really exciting thing. Pert believes that if the mind is defined as brain cells communicating with one another then, since peptides and their receptors are in the body as well as in the brain (where they're called neuropeptides), then the mind is in the body. In fact, the body *is* the unconscious mind.

What's more, according to Pert, in virtually all locations where information from any of the five senses enters the nervous system, there's always a high concentration of neuropeptide receptors. These regions are known as nodal points or, more colloquially, hot spots, because they're places where a great deal of information converges (Molecules of Emotion, 1999).

Are these nodal points chakras? They certainly could be. That would tie in with the concept that chakras exist not just in a handful of special places, but whenever and wherever the unconscious mind is in a process of transformation. Especially when an altered state of consciousness is created.

The chakras and their symbols

The symbols used for the principal chakras have evolved over centuries and become more and more elaborate. Different schools of Tantra use different symbols on which to meditate, but here I present a system that is widely recognized.

Muladhara chakra. *Muladhara* means 'root support' and is situated at the base of the spine. This chakra is, as it were, the 'switch' for engorgement of the erectile tissues. Its symbols are: a yellow square (representing Earth); the royal elephant Airavata with seven trunks (representing the potential to awaken the other six principal and 'sub' chakras); a five-headed Lord Brahma sitting upon the elephant's head; **Dakini,** mistress of the skin, seated to Brahma's right; *Kundalini* coiled three-and-a-half times round the 'Shiva *Lingam*'; the mantra *Lam* (pronounced 'lung').

Swadhisthana chakra. *Swadhisthana* means 'one's own place' and is situated a short distance up the spine, just below the navel. This chakra controls the sexual fluids. Its symbols are: a white crescent (representing the moon); the fire-breathing crocodile known as Makara; the god **Vishnu,** the preserver of life; the two-headed goddess

(Contd)

Rakini, who grants the power of sex magic; the mantra *Vam* (pronounced 'vung').

Manipura chakra. *Manipura* means 'jewel city' and is situated at the level of the solar plexus. This chakra controls passion. Its symbols are: a red triangle (representing the *yoni*); the ram Mesha (battering down all obstacles); the god Rudra, Lord of the tears of passion; Lakini, ruler of all flesh; the mantra *Ram* (pronounced 'rung').

Anahata chakra. *Anahata* means 'unstruck sound' and is situated at the level of the heart. Its symbols are: blue interlocking triangles (representing union); an antelope (representing sensitivity); the god **Indra** (representing the power of the *lingam*); the four-headed goddess Kakini; the mantra *Yam* (pronounced 'yung').

Vishuddhi chakra. *Vishuddhi* means 'with purity' and is located at the base of the throat. This chakra is specifically concerned with the transformation of sexual energy into *Soma* or *Amrita*, the 'elixir of the gods'. Its symbols are: a full white moon against a blue background; the five-headed Sadashiva, Lord of transformation; the five-headed Shakini, representing the 'lower' senses; an albino elephant; the mantra *Ham* (pronounced 'hung').

Ajna chakra. *Ajna* means 'command centre' and is located in the middle of the forehead, just above the level of the eyebrows. This chakra is the 'third eye'. Its symbols are the androgynous deity Paramshiva emerging from a phallic thumb; the six-headed goddess Hakini, representing the five senses plus intuition: the mantra **OM** (pronounced 'aah-oh-ong'). When all the lower chakras have opened, the energy should automatically open the *Ajna* chakra and the next one.

Sahasrara chakra. This is a very special kind of chakra known as the thousand-petalled lotus. It's the ultimate level of bliss. When *Kundalini* reaches the *Sahasrara* it's the end of the journey. Only when *Kundalini* has ascended many times will she stay permanently. The Tantrika then becomes, in the words of the *Sat-Cakra-Nirupana*, 'all joy, and is the Eternal itself'.

The 'ng' sound at the end of the mantras is made with the mouth open and is not a closed-mouthed, humming 'mmm'. For a full explanation of how to pronounce *OM* see Chapter 4.

THE POWER OF THE MIND IN TANTRIC SEX

What we can say for certain about chakras is that whether or not they exist in any form at all, they were used, and can be used by you, as meditative tools in Tantric sex for the achievement of *ananda*.

Traditionally, the male Tantrika would first of all sit in the lotus position and perform a rite to, as it were, connect himself with the Earth. Meditating on the *Muladhara* chakra he would then draw his Shakti onto his lap, awakening *Kundalini*. As sex progressed, so *Kundalini* would be forced to uncurl and enter the bottom of the *susumna nadi* (in or beside the spine) and the Tantrika would endeavour to drive the energy higher and higher, meditating on each chakra as it was reached. If he was skilful and dedicated enough, he would eventually 'pierce' the fifth chakra, causing the sixth (*Ajna*) and seventh (*Sahasrara*) to open automatically. The result would be *samadhi*, or enlightenment or, to put it in more Western terms, the ultimate ecstasy.

As I've said, Tantric sex was originally about men using women, which is why I referred to the *sadhaka* as 'he'. But, interestingly, we have direct scientific evidence not only of the effectiveness of this style of meditation but of its effectiveness specifically in women. A team led by Beverly Whipple of Rutgers University, New Jersey, studied ten women who could orgasm by thought alone. They were monitored both when masturbating and when arousing themselves entirely by the power of their minds. In both styles, heart rate, blood pressure, pupil dilation and pain threshold approximately doubled, so there's no doubting the genuineness of the mind-induced orgasms. Some of the women thought of erotic scenes, but others visualized *energy ascending and descending the spine*. That, effectively, is what Tantrikas do.

The ten women in the Rutgers study were, of course, exceptional. They needed no physical stimulation to reach orgasm. Almost certainly you will. But let's find out how far you (woman or man) can go by, like them, using only the power of your mind to create sexual excitement and then to drive it up into your brain to alter your state of consciousness.

Have a go
- ▶ Step 1: *Undress and sit or lie somewhere comfortable.*
- ▶ Step 2: *Call up your favourite sexual fantasy.*
- ▶ Step 3: *Once you've generated some excitement, perform* **vajroli mudra** *(see Chapter 8) while imagining the energy being drawn up your spine into your brain and, as it were, pouring onto your fantasy like petrol on a fire, making it even more vivid and intense. You may find it helps to suck in air through your mouth in short sips.*
- ▶ Step 4: *Check your degree of physical excitement (erection/ wetness) and mental excitement.*

TRANSFORMING SEXUAL ENERGY

Now let's see what you can achieve *with* physical excitement. We're going to use visualizations during masturbation. You can visualize the established Tantric chakras if you prefer (see the chakras factbox, p. 31) but they were designed for the Eastern mind and, although it's claimed they're part of the collective unconscious of the human race, probably won't mean very much to you. You'll almost certainly do better by creating your own visualizations. Neuro-Linguistic Programming has taken this process to a whole new level (see the NLP factbox, pp. 36–38).

Have a go

▶ **Step 1:** *Create your own chakra symbols. You don't have to have an official number of chakras and, for simplicity, I suggest starting with just three (let's say the* Muladhara, *the* Anahata *and the* Ajna) *and seeing how that works. Remember, we're looking for a gradual transformation of raw sexual energy into* ananda, *so the symbols should progressively reflect that. If you're a man then you would probably locate your first chakra in your* lingam *(approximately the* Muladhara *chakra). Your visualization might then be your partner opening her thighs to reveal a bright red* yoni *while, as a mantra, she incites you to do all the things you've ever wanted. If you're a woman you'd probably locate your first chakra in your* yoni *and visualize being penetrated by your lover. For both men and women, the second chakra might be located at the heart (*Anahata *chakra) and the visualization might be, say, running towards one another in slow-motion through a carpet of sunlit autumn leaves to the sound of your favourite romantic song. Your final chakra (*Ajna) *would be located in your brain and your visualization would be the kind of spiritual experience that you're seeking – it could be floating through space with your partner, your soul uniting with your partner's soul, arriving in Paradise, or whatever accords with your hopes and beliefs.*

▶ **Step 2:** *Spend time every day running through your visualizations, improving them in every way you can. Eventually you should be able to call them to mind in vivid detail.*

▶ **Step 3:** *Choose an occasion when you have plenty of time and won't be disturbed. Undress and arouse yourself in your usual way.*

▶ **Step 4:** *Call up your first visualization (which will be the most erotic), while continuing to stimulate yourself physically. You may find it helps to speak out loud the 'mantra' (the sexy things you or your partner would be saying).*

▶ **Step 5:** *Once you've (hopefully) aroused* Kundalini, *imagine sucking the energy up towards your* Anahata *chakra. It will* *probably help to pull in your stomach while noisily sucking air in through your mouth in small sips.*

▶ **Step 6:** *Call up your second visualization and dwell on it while increasing physical stimulation. Remember that at this stage you're trying to transmute the sexual energy into love.*

▶ **Step 7:** *Overwhelmed by feelings of love, imagine the energy once again being sucked upwards, this time to the* Ajna *chakra.*

▶ **Step 8:** *Call up your third visualization and dwell on it as you increase physical stimulation even more and approach orgasm/ejaculation.*

▶ **Step 9:** *You started with sexual energy. You changed it into love. Now you're transforming love into* ananda. *Linger there. Stay right on the edge as long as possible.*

▶ **Step 10:** *The eventual aim is that you should be flooded with* rasa-*juice, but you have a bit more reading to do before that stage is reached. For now you can either orgasm/ejaculate or allow the energy to die away on its own.*

Insight

I find it much easier to call up photographs or films than actual scenes from real life – perhaps just because I can take plenty of time studying an image. So when I want to be able to visualize something that's very important, I take a digital photograph and view it on my computer. Or I watch a scene on a DVD over and over again and then, in my imagination, substitute myself and my partner in place of the actors.

NLP and chakras

Neuro-Linguistic Programming (NLP) provides a whole set of tools for getting into your unconscious mind in a way that, for most people, will be far more powerful than the traditional chakras. The ones we're particularly interested in are visualization and anchoring.

Of course, we all use visualization. But most of us are not very good at it. In NLP-type visualization you'll use every technique of the modern cinema (plus a few more) as if you're an Oscar-winning film director. Let's say you want to arouse yourself by thinking of something sexy. First of all, call up your visualization and play around with the colours, the size, the sound quality and so on (what in NLP are called 'submodalities') to achieve the effect you want. Then get really creative for maximum impact. Here are some ideas:

▶ *See the scene through your own eyes.*
▶ *Now switch 'cameras' to see the scene from another person's viewpoint.*
▶ *Pull back to see everyone in the scene simultaneously.*
▶ *Make a split screen and show different images side by side.*
▶ *Run a section in slow motion.*
▶ *Show a series of stills.*
▶ *Change 'camera angles'.*
▶ *Play some music.*
▶ *Play some completely different music.*
▶ *Use soft focus.*
▶ *Introduce a voiceover.*
▶ *Zoom in for a close-up.*
▶ *Move in closer still.*
▶ *Pull right back so you can now see for miles.*
▶ *Turn down the lights.*
▶ *Switch from colour to black and white.*

Don't worry if you can't actually see an image very clearly or for very long. That's how it is for most people. If you practise regularly you will get better. And as this is all in your mind you can do a few things Hollywood can't yet achieve, such as use scent, taste and texture.

Anchors have always existed as part of the human mind and have been exploited for thousands of years, but once again

(Contd)

NLP has taken them to a new level. An anchor is simply something that triggers an automatic behaviour or mindset. The example that's usually given is the brake light on the rear of a car. Once you've learned to drive, the illumination of a brake light on a car ahead will make you move your foot to your brake pedal without any conscious thought being involved. The same is true for all religious and spiritual rituals – the words and objects used are, basically, anchors. With repetition they automatically and instantly engender the right mental state.

We can take this principle and adapt it for Tantric sex. Whenever you're masturbating, play music that evokes spiritual thoughts and feelings in you. Conjure up spiritual images rather than sexual images. And use accessories that have a spiritual significance – incense, for example. As a result, over time you'll come to associate sex quite automatically with spiritual feelings.

IS KUNDALINI DANGEROUS?

There are various views of *Kundalini*. According to one school of Tantra, as described by Pandit R. Anantakrsna Sastri, *Kundalini* is something quite distinct and lies dormant in most people throughout their lives. In this school, the piercing of the chakras is not a rapid and temporary phenomenon but a gradual ascent over many years. A person who dies at a particular stage is reincarnated at that stage and proceeds from there. That's not the view I take.

According to another school of thought, as described by Swamiji Satyananda in *Tantra of Kundaline Yoga*, awakening can take place in 'one month, three months, in one day'. But the problem is that a 'weak mind' cannot 'sustain the terrible force of the flow of Shakti'. The result is that 12 years are necessary, not for the awakening, but 'to prepare yourself to hold the awakening'.

My personal view is that we all awaken *Kundalini* but most of us just don't raise her very far. In fact, there is a condition known as *Kundalini* Syndrome and a not insignificant number of people claim to have suffered it including, most famously, the Indian mystic Gopi Krishna (1903–84), who described how at the age of 34, after 17 years of meditation, 'something exploded in my brain and a current of silvery light rising from my spine radiated throughout my whole brain, and I felt myself expanding in all directions.' He then went through various crises until, at the age of 49, the transformation process was complete and he lived 'in two different worlds', a world of normal perception and a world in which he saw consciousness in everything as if it were living – in the sea, in a mountain, in the sky, in the Earth itself. His explanation is that he had activated a normally dormant region of the brain known as **Brahmarendra** (cavity of Brahman), thus gaining the same vision of the universe 'that all mystics have'.

Westerners who say they've suffered *Kundalini* Syndrome describe the symptoms as including sensitivity to light and sound, cramps, rapid pulse, headaches and anxiety, none of which are desirable but all of which could be due to many things. They also talk of strange currents running up the spine, which is more difficult to account for. And they complain of genital tingling, mystical experiences and a feeling of being out of touch with reality.

I interviewed one man about why he had stopped practising Tantric sex. 'We now have two children and my wife is often tired,' he explained. 'You need time for Tantric sex because it becomes the whole focus of your life.'

This is the more likely impact of *Kundalini*. You'll have 'sex on the brain' and you need to have a regular partner who is just as interested as you are. If you've been reading this book alone, stop now and involve your partner.

A final word of advice. Don't meditate on things you don't truly want. If day after day, month after month, you meditate on the visible universe as an illusion then, inevitably, you will at some stage, by definition, become divorced from 'reality'.

> ### Insight
> I personally recognize the 'genital tingling', the 'mystical feelings' and the sense of being 'out of touch with reality', if that means seeing life somewhat differently to the way most people do. And I count them as positives. I *like* to feel the electric current of constant desire for my partner. I like talking to flowers. And I like the fact that Tantric sex has changed my priorities and my way of looking at the world.

10 THINGS TO REMEMBER

1 *You can focus energy in different parts of your own body.*

2 *You can send energy to your partner and receive energy from your partner.*

3 *Tantrikas believe there's a special source of energy at the base of the spine, envisaged as a snake goddess called* Kundalini *(in the Hindu tradition) or* Candalini *(in the Buddhist tradition) who seeks union with the god Shiva who dwells in the brain.*

4 *The real source of energy in the human body is not a snake but billions of 'bugs' called mitochondria; nevertheless, Western science has described a 'gland' that might be connected with the* Kundalini *story.*

5 *Tantrikas believe that in addition to the physical body, everyone also possesses a 'subtle body' in which there are* nadis *or energy channels; some Western scientists believe the recently discovered system of neuropeptides may correspond with the 'subtle body'.*

6 *Tantric sex techniques are designed to arouse* Kundalini *and drive her upwards along the* sushumna nadi, *which follows the spine.*

7 *As* Kundalini *rises, Tantrikas meditate on a series of chakras so as to transform the raw sexual energy into spiritual energy.*

8 *Rather than using traditional chakra symbols, you can instead use modern visualization and anchoring techniques.*

9 *Beverly Whipple of Rutgers University, New Jersey, studied women who could orgasm from thought alone, including some whose technique was to envisage energy moving up and down the spine, much as Tantrikas do.*

10 *It's important to have a partner who is as interested in Tantric sex as you are, otherwise the sexual energy you generate will not have an outlet.*

HOW TANTRIC ARE YOU NOW?

- ☐ Have you successfully raised the temperature of your hands?
- ☐ By focusing your mind, have you been able to direct energy to various parts of your body?
- ☐ Have you been able to send energy to different parts of your partner's body?
- ☐ Has your partner been able to send energy to different parts of your body?
- ☐ Have you begun a regular exercise programme for your PC muscle?
- ☐ Have you been able to arouse yourself entirely through the power of your mind?
- ☐ Have you either created your own chakra symbols or memorized the traditional ones?
- ☐ Have you been able to transform your sexual energy into spiritual energy?
- ☐ Have you tried using modern NLP techniques to help you?
- ☐ Have you involved your partner in learning about Tantric sex?

If you answered 'yes' to between eight and ten questions you're obviously very open to Tantric sex ideas and have worked hard on acquiring the skills.

If you answered 'yes' to between five and seven questions you're on your way but you have quite a bit of experimenting and practising to do.

If you couldn't answer 'yes' to more than four questions, read the chapter again and really get down to training your mind and your body. It's the most fun you'll ever have learning new things.

3

....

Breaking taboos

In this chapter you will learn:
- *why you should discard your inhibitions and how*
- *the Tantric 'Five Ms'*
- *the secrets of the* cakrapuja.

> *The Tantrika should never drink the wine meant for the*
> *goddess, unless the same has first been offered to her.*
> *Drinking should only be continued so long as the mind is*
> *absorbed in the goddess.*
>
> *Tantraraja Tantra*

The breaking of taboos was, and remains, an important part of
Tantric sex. The idea was that if you wanted to expand your
consciousness you had to overthrow old ways of thinking and escape
the boundaries set by mere humans. For the gods (and the aim was
to become a god) there were no rules and nothing was wrong.

This sentiment is known in other cultures, too. An Arab saying,
often quoted by Sir Richard Burton, the Victorian explorer and
co-translator of the *Kama Sutra*, is 'To the pure all things are pure'.
It's a concept we can grasp intuitively, as long as it's not taken to
an extreme. For example, we can easily see that there are actions
that could be 'pure' or 'impure' depending on motivation. To have
sex with a willing partner with a feeling of love is clearly 'pure'
while to have sex with the same person in the same way while
pretending love is 'impure'.

But there's also another aspect of this breaking of taboos. If you're going to reach the highest raptures of Tantric sex it's essential you should rid yourself of all inhibitions. You can't, as it were, mingle body with body, soul with soul, spirit with spirit, if you're going to hold back. You have to be totally accessible to your partner and your partner has to be totally accessible to you. That may mean doing things you've never done before.

Essentially you have to view your body as a tool, a tool of the spirit. As with any tool you have to look after it but you also have to be willing to use it to the full to achieve the end for which, in the Tantric view, it was designed. That is to say, to unleash the maximum sexual energy for the achievement of the highest level of *ananda*.

Insight

Some commentators have expressed concern about Tantric sex being used as an excuse for exploitation. I would argue that in consensual Tantric sex between two people who love one another, the man is the god, the woman is the goddess, and the things that are done are beyond ordinary banalities to do with who puts what where, for how long and so forth. That's too trivial. That's not to say you shouldn't have any 'rules' at all. But it does mean you shouldn't blindly accept society's conventions, or things you were told by your parents, or were taught at school or by a religious instructor. You need to question why you 'can't' do certain things and why you 'should' do other things. If the answers stand up to scrutiny, that's fine. But if they don't then maybe that's a 'taboo' you should break.

The Five Ms

The offerings that Tantrikas used in their sexualized rituals have changed in number and type over the centuries, and from culture to culture. According to Edward Sellon (1818–1866), an English army officer who served in India and who wrote *Annotations Upon the*

Sacred Writings of the Hindus (1865), those in his time were 'flesh, fish, wine, women, and certain mystical twisting or gesticulations with the fingers'. And according to the Reverend William Ward, a clergyman based in India, they were 'broiled fish, flesh, fried peas, rice, spirituous liquors, sweetmeats, flowers, and other offerings...'

But the most common were the Five Makaras or 'Five Ms', so-called because each begins with the letter 'M' in the Sanskrit language (*mudra, madhya, matsya, mamsa, maithuna*). Their use was also known as the Tantric Great Rite of the Five Essentials or the *Pancha Makara* – *pancha* means 'five' and *makara* is the name of a mythical beast which was a combination of various creatures. All of the five, according to many authorities, were taboo.

MUDRA – *AN APHRODISIAC?*

Mudra is translated in many books on Tantra as grain or cereal and, indeed, the *Yogini Tantra* clearly says that 'all such cereals as are chewed are called *Mudra*'. However, grain never was a taboo so either the Five Ms weren't necessarily taboos after all (a view held by some) or the translation is wrong. In fact, *mudra* can also be translated as 'seal', a euphemism for the vulva, which could make sense, because as we'll see in Chapter 6, the drinking of sexual fluids either directly from the vulva or from a cup or bowl was an important part of Tantric ritual. Yet another possible translation is 'gesture' and it's clear from Edward Sellon's account that special hand movements were part of the ceremony at one time. But my personal view is that the original meaning in this context was an aphrodisiac prepared from grain. We know that in the Ancient Greek fertility ritual known as the *thesmophoria*, women drank *kykeon* in order to receive transcendent visions. It seems very likely that it was derived from ergot, a fungus that grows on barley and which causes hallucinations. So that, or something like it, is a possibility. The seeds of datura (jimson weed), still used by Tantrikas today to induce trance, are another.

Nowadays we have some extremely strong drugs available for sex but they should only be prescribed by a doctor after a medical check-up. Do not self-medicate with drugs bought on the internet. Some natural products work but generally need to be taken for some time before they have an effect. They include ginkgo biloba (which improves blood circulation to the genitals), garlic (which does the same), saw palmetto (which, for men, increases 'free' testosterone), zinc (which increases testosterone in men who had been zinc-deficient) and maca. Why not buy a 'sex tonic' at a health food shop and try it?

But we're really interested here in exciting sexual desire through the breaking of taboos. So if there are things you know your partner would like you to do but which you've rejected, take some time to reconsider. Why not play with a vibrator? Why not put on that sexy underwear or that fireman's outfit? Why not shave your pubic hair? Why not act dominant or submissive for a little while? If you don't really have a good reason, get rid of that taboo.

MADHYA – *WINE*

Madhya is wine. It was also known as *vama-amrta* or 'nectar-of-the-left' because the left stood for things that were abnormal or forbidden (see *maithuna* below). According to the *Mahanirvana Tantra* it should ideally be served in a *pana patra* (cup) of gold, silver or glass. Tantrikas who were less well off might have used a coconut and some drank from a skull, partly for the shock value and partly as a reminder that death awaits everyone.

How much wine did Tantrikas drink during sex? Some scholars argue that alcohol was only sipped as a symbolic gesture, as in Communion. Others say the Tantrikas became completely drunk to help them overcome their inhibitions about public sex (see below) and to enter all the more easily into an altered state of consciousness. So what's the evidence?

According to Abbé Jean-Antoine Dubois, a Frenchman who lived in India for some 30 years around the beginning of the nineteenth century, the Tantrikas drank to get drunk. In his *Moeurs, Institutions et Cérémonies des Peuples de l'Inde*

(Manners, Customs and Ceremonies of the Indian People, 1825) he wrote that 'everyone became intoxicated drinking from the bowl in turn' and that when they were 'completely drunk' men and women 'mingled freely for the rest of the night'. Critics say the abbé never witnessed these things himself but his account is confirmed by a later European, Elizabeth Sharpe, who wrote a book called *The Secrets of the Kaula Circle* (1936), *Kaula* being a sect within Tantra:

> *Man after man, woman after woman passed me by, singing, reeling and dead drunk... I, still, remember that inner courtyard: stark naked men and women, who, from time to time, with excruciating yells, leapt to their feet, shaking their heads backwards and forwards, the women with loosened locks falling in black disorder about their heaving, shaking breasts. A voice would then cry out in deepest scorn the sonorous Sanskrit Tantrik verse: 'Let their desires be satisfied.' And there would be a perfect orgy of bestiality.*

Those who say these writers were prejudiced need only refer to the ancient texts. The c. eleventh century *Kulacudamani Tantra* says the guru should be naked, with betel leaf in his mouth (see the factbox, pp. 48–9), his hair hanging free, and his eyes rolling 'from the effect of wine'. The twelfth or thirteenth century *Rudrayamala* talks of naked semi-divine *Siddhas* 'having sex with beautiful women, all of them red-eyed, stuffed full, and drunk on meat and alcohol'. And the tenth century *Tantraloka* of **Abhinavagupta** is quite clear that without alcohol 'there is neither enjoyment nor liberation'.

A balanced Western view was provided by Alexandra David-Néel in her book *L'Inde Que J'ai Connue* (*The India I Knew*, 1951). Daringly she hid so that she could watch a Tantric ceremony and reported that it was a 'truly religious' act. 'It is known,' she concluded, 'that other shaktas in other similar gatherings wallow in drunken orgies, this is known and I have watched this in Nepal, but this was not the case in this particular unknown house.'

And that really sums it up. Some Tantrikas drank a little wine, some drank rather more (but, as it advises in the *Kulacudamani*

Tantra, kept their senses 'under control'), and others went in for binge drinking.

Betel and *soma*

But it wasn't just wine. There were other drugs involved as well, including cannabis, and especially betel or *pan*, still widely used in Asia today, where couples chew and exchange it from mouth to mouth as foreplay, creating blood-red saliva. The ancient symbolism is clear, standing for menstrual blood and the blood produced by a virgin's first intercourse.

Betel is a mixture of leaves and nuts from two different plants (and sometimes additional flavourings, too). According to mythology, the discovery of the combined effect came about when a strange creeper was found growing in an urn in which *amrut* (the equivalent of the Greek ambrosia, the food of the gods) had been stored. The god Vishnu was curious and, as a result, the intriguing minty/peppery taste of betel was discovered. In reality, the betel creeper grows on the areca tree (*Areca Catechu*) which resembles the coconut palm and produces huge clusters of hazel-sized nuts. The leaf can be chewed alone but it was inevitable that someone would find out what would happen when the nuts and the leaves were eaten together. The answer is: quite a lot. Westerners who try *pan* for the first time report a powerful effect. They feel more alert and more vigorous to the point of euphoria, hot, sweaty and sexually aroused. For maximum effect lime powder can be added (from cooking coral over a bonfire for several days) together with various aromatics to improve the flavour (such as cardamom, camphor, tobacco or nutmeg). The wealthy used ground pearls in place of coral, together with whipped butter and saffron.

That betel was an important part of Tantric ritual is clear from numerous texts. The *Kaulajnananirnaya* of

Matsyendranatha, for example, talks of a Shakti 'garlanded by sky' (that is, naked) with her hair hanging loose and her mouth smeared with tambula (betel leaf). And according to the sixteenth century *Kaulavalinirnaya* of Jnanananda Paramahamsa, a Shiva should chew betel before uniting *lingam* and *yoni*.

It seems that a drink called *soma* may also sometimes have been used, in the belief that it bestowed divine qualities. In the *Rig Veda* (the Hindu 'Bible') there is a line that 'we have drunk *soma* and become immortal'. We know the drink was prepared by a priest pounding a plant with a stone but we don't know what that plant was. Some scholars have put forward the hallucinogenic fly agaric (*Amanita muscaria*) but, in the quantities it seems to have been drunk, fly agaric would have been fatal. My belief is that *soma* was prepared from a species of Ephedra, which was still being used by Zoroatrians in Iran in the nineteenth century to make a drink they called *homa*. *Homa* acts like adrenaline, which fits in with *soma* also having been drunk before battle.

Have a go

So what, if anything, should you take? Dietary supplements containing Ephedra were banned by the US Food and Drug Administration (FDA) in 2004. Betel stains the teeth permanently and horribly and, anyway, isn't available outside Asia. And I certainly couldn't advocate the use of marijuana or other illegal drugs. As regards alcohol, any large quantity limits both sensation and response. The sex might *seem* more exciting but, in reality – in terms of degree of erection, wetness, hormones and so on – it isn't.

I'm not going to encourage you to take up alcohol if you don't drink it now. But if you do drink alcohol then I would suggest the following:

▶ **Step 1:** *Choose a container that will create a sense of occasion for you. It could be a very nice wine glass. Whatever it is, keep* *it exclusively for your Tantric ritual and don't use it on any other occasion.*

▶ **Step 2:** *With ceremony, pour a little wine into the container and share it between you, passing the container back and forth, a sip at a time, while you gaze into one another's eyes. For more intimacy, take some wine into your own mouth and kiss it into your partner's mouth.*

▶ **Step 3:** *Replenish your container with a little wine. Make love in the Tantric style, as explained in this book and, at suitable moments* during lovemaking, *again share wine.*

▶ **Step 4:** *When you've finished your lovemaking, replenish the container a third time and share it as before.*

Insight

The best time to drink alcohol (if you drink it at all) is, in fact, *afterwards* when your brains will be awash with dopamine. The wine will then have the effect of prolonging that dopamine 'hit' by effectively slowing its re-uptake. Dopamine is a pleasure-giving neurotransmitter and contributes to the post-coital glow. However, if you always accompany sex with alcohol, also try it without. Alcohol lowers a chemical called oxytocin, which is responsible for skin pleasure and your orgasmic contractions (for more on this, see Chapter 5).

MATSYA *AND* MAMSA – *FISH AND MEAT*

Matsya is fish and *mamsa* is meat. Strict Hindus eat neither, firstly because of the Dharmic (religious) law of *ahinsa* or non-injury which, in the Vedic scripture, is an obligation to the gods. According to the *Mahabharata*, the epic Sanskrit poem, *ahinsa* is 'the highest Dharma...the highest self-control...the highest teaching... He who desires to augment his own flesh by eating the flesh of other creatures lives in misery.' Secondly, eating meat is said to lead to 'karmic bondage' – that's to say, the suffering someone causes to animals will in turn be suffered by that person in a future incarnation. Thirdly, there is a belief that if you eat the flesh of animals so you also consume their emotions and lower consciousness. After the Muslim invasion and, later, the British invasion, many Hindus did convert to the foreign way of eating but, for strict Hindus in early Tantric ritual, breaking the taboo about *matsya* and *mamsa* would, indeed, have been significant. If that wasn't already enough, the *Kaulajnananirnaya* of Matsyendranatha says that followers should eat jackal, dog and other 'impure creatures' to increase the shock value. That philosophy is confirmed by Jayaratha in his commentary to the *Tantraloka* which says that *viras* (heroes) should eat what ordinary men detest and which is prohibited by the scriptures.

For us in the West today, probably the key element to be preserved in this is not so much the food itself but the ritual that surrounded it. The food was passed from mouth to mouth, a tremendous act of intimacy designed to create a collective consciousness.

Have a go

▶ **Step 1:** *Choose a container that will create a sense of occasion for you. It could be a very nice ceramic bowl, for example. Whatever it is, keep it exclusively for your Tantric ritual and don't use it on any other occasion.*

▶ **Step 2:** *Prepare some suitable food and arrange it in the bowl. Choose things you don't normally eat and that are particularly tangy or piquant. Examples might be unusual nuts (such as macadamias), unusual fruits (such as cumquats), Indian delicacies such as onion bhajees, Middle Eastern snacks such as falafels, or sweets such as Turkish delights.*

▶ **Step 3:** *Before sex, after sex and during sex, pass an item of food back and forth between your mouths, sucking and chewing it until it's gone.*

Insight

If you are a vegetarian or vegan, I don't think you'd be expanding your consciousness by eating meat. On the other hand, if you are a meat eater you might well find you expand your consciousness by trying to be a vegetarian or vegan for a time. That will be far more conducive to becoming part of the 'great Oneness'. What's more, avoiding the saturated fats in meat will help maintain a healthy blood flow to your erectile tissues.

MAITHUNA – *SEX*

Maithuna means sex. But, of course, sex isn't now and never was a taboo. So what kind of sex are we talking about? The answer is group sex. I won't be suggesting you take part. However, Tantric sex as described in this book is an adaptation of the ideas and techniques used in the sexualized rituals of the Tantric sect called the *Kaula*, and it's essential to know about them if you want to have a good understanding of what you're doing and why.

It's already clear from the eyewitness accounts that the *Kaula* rituals took various forms. When you keep in mind that Tantra has been embraced by various cultures over many centuries without ever having any central authority, it could never have been any other way. It's impossible to point to any particular manner of doing things and say that that's the 'true path'.

The *Kaula* sect is usually divided into two groups, those who followed the left-hand path (*vama*) and those who followed the right-hand path (*daksina*). Some say the names come from the fact that the left side of the body was considered female and that the female was considered more sexual, while the right was considered male. Others say that when those involved in the rituals were going to have sex the woman sat to the man's left, whereas if sex wasn't involved the woman sat to the man's right. Yet other authorities say the right-hand path could involve sex, but only between a husband and his wife (*Adya Shakti*), whereas the left-hand path involved sex between a man and a woman who was his partner for the night only (*Svakiya Shakti*). In practice, there never was a sharp division. There were Tantrikas who never took part in sex rituals at all, there were those who sometimes took part in 'right-handed' sex ceremonies and sometimes in 'left-handed', and there were those who followed the left-hand path exclusively. What's clear is that the left-hand path was more extreme, sometimes very, very extreme and has been likened by many Hindus to black magic and witchcraft.

But why *group* sex? The answer is to create a group consciousness. In some cases this had a very worldly, practical application and in others an otherworldly goal. The worldly goal was to bind the participants together as a clan or *kula*. The otherworldly goal, the one we're more interested in, was to dissolve the ego and experience oneness with a small group of people. As a couple, you can learn something from that and adapt the ideas to your own private bedroom, seeking oneness between yourselves.

The *Pancatattva* or 'secret ritual' usually took the form of men and women sitting alternately in a circle, when it was known as *cakrapuja* or *chakra puja* (*cakra/chakra* means circle, *puja* means worship). If the participants were not going to have sex with their own spouses one method of selection was the notorious *cudacakra* in which women put their jackets (*cuda*) in a pile and each man selected one. The men and women could therefore be from completely different castes, another aspect of breaking taboo. The couples would then be ritually wedded for the night, with the man asking something like, 'Do you elect me as your husband for this ritual?' If the woman accepted she would offer flowers and rice, and place her hands in his, and the two of them would sprinkle water on the guru.

Everything was preceded by the most elaborate and lengthy ceremonies which had to be carried out precisely and in the prescribed way. Even when physical contact had begun, there was a lengthy kind of 'foreplay' known as *nyasa* (see Chapter 5) which involved touching, massaging and stimulating different parts of the body and identifying them, through mantras (see Chapter 4), with the body of the god or goddess. For each part of the body participants would first recite a mantra:

> *Ang, Kring, Kring, Yang, Rang, Lang, Vang, Shang, Shang, Sang, Hong, Haung, Hangsah.*

And then follow that by saying something like, 'The embodied spirit of the highly blessed and auspicious *Kalika* is placed here.'

The importance of having the right mental attitude is made clear by the tenth century *Tantraloka* of Abhinavagupta, which says that no one should be allowed to enter the circle for the wrong reasons because they will then destroy the pleasure of expansive consciousness.

Alexandra David-Néel (see p. 47) described what she saw like this:

> *A long time elapsed, and then each worshipper drew his shakti against his body... Each Tantrist had only one shakti, either his spouse or his shakti chosen for one night only. Of course, it was impossible to guess what kind of relationship existed between the couples I saw. To me, the fifth part of the puja or the ritualistic intercourse, appeared to be perfectly chaste... The sadhakas remained silent and motionless like those sculptures of Hindu gods embracing their goddesses, performing a truly religious act, devoid of any obscenity.*

Such icy control was even more essential for the rite known as *anandabhuvana-yoga* in which a *vira* would have sex with anything from three to 108 women. Some scholars say that all but one of the women would merely have been touched but using the techniques to prevent ejaculation described in Chapters 7 and 8, it's quite possible to have intercourse with a large number of women. It may have happened.

Have a go

Most couples will not want to take part in *cakra puja*. But given that it was the quintessential ritual within Tantric sex, is it really possible to have genuine Tantric sex without it? In my opinion, yes. You can still use the physical techniques to enjoy the most exciting sex of your life. And you can still use the mental techniques to forge a profound sense of oneness with your partner and with the cosmos. What isn't possible is to generate that sense of a collective consciousness together with others in the circle and thus to create a clan or *kula* of people bound together by their experience.

So what can you do? One possibility, which might involve breaking a taboo for you, could be to go to a nudist beach and simply enjoy the sense of community that comes from being naked together with other people. Another idea might be to play an erotic DVD while making love (see Erotica on p. 62).

Tantra in the mind

Not all followers of Tantra took part in the sexualized rituals. Some concentrated entirely on other techniques of consciousness expansion such as meditation and mantra. And some had sex just in the mind. In fact, achieving *samadhi* entirely by internal processes was considered to be the highest level of attainment.

For example, instead of drinking alcohol or taking drugs, some flooded their brains with 'nectar' entirely by the power of thought – that's to say, with the body's natural opiates or endorphins. Instead of eating meat they 'ate' their own tongues, a practice known as *Khechari Mudra*. And *Khechari Mudra* also served in place of intercourse, with the tongue representing the *lingam*, the soft palate the clitoris, and the nasal-pharynx the *yoni*. A man would stretch out the tongue and flick it from side to side across the front teeth so that, after a few weeks, the lingual frenum attaching the tongue to the floor of the mouth, would be partially worn away. He could then insert his substitute penis into his substitute vagina (and, apparently, also stick it out and up to the eyebrows). You may prefer to remain at the 'lower' *Kaula* level, using a real *lingam* and a real *yoni*.

I certainly wouldn't recommend doing anything to damage the lingual frenum in any way. The tongue is, however, an important tool in Tantric sex in far more approachable ways, as we'll see in Chapter 6.

Breaking your personal taboos

None of the 'five Ms' are taboo in our society other than group or public sex. So if you want to celebrate the dynamism of the universe you're going to have to find some other 'forbidden fruits' that you can symbolically enjoy. What can you do?

Let's find out what your inhibitions are. Here's a little quiz; tick the answers you agree with.

I'm not at all inhibited about:
- [ ] undressing in front of my partner.
- [ ] sleeping naked with my partner.
- [ ] showering or bathing with my partner.
- [ ] being naked on the beach.
- [ ] talking about sex with my partner.
- [ ] telling my partner exactly what I want him/her to do sexually.
- [ ] telling my partner my sexual fantasies.
- [ ] making love in full light.
- [ ] my partner knowing I masturbate.
- [ ] my partner watching me masturbate.
- [ ] 'talking dirty' during sex.
- [ ] trying new sex techniques and positions.
- [ ] making love in different places.
- [ ] using a mirror or camera to increase arousal.
- [ ] using pornography to increase arousal.
- [ ] how I look when I orgasm.
- [ ] how much noise I make when I orgasm.
- [ ] my partner seeing my genitals.
- [ ] my partner seeing my anus.
- [ ] using any part of my body for sexual pleasure.

So how did you get on? Since you're reading this book it's unlikely you made fewer than five ticks but if you did then you need to get to work on those inhibitions. You may find you need professional help, especially if your anxieties are connected with some earlier trauma. If you scored six to ten ticks you're still quite inhibited but you can probably improve with the help of this book alone. If you scored 11 to 15 ticks, you're already fairly uninhibited and can easily become more so. If you scored 16 or more ticks, you're obviously extremely uninhibited and well on your way to becoming a Tantrika.

Both you and your partner need to be uninhibited if you're going to explore Tantric sex to the full. But there's one consolation if you are inhibited, and that's the fun you're going to have breaking your taboos.

Being uninhibited doesn't mean doing things you don't want to do. It means doing things you do want to do but that you've been afraid to do. And it means doing them without feeling guilty. If you can't be yourself with your partner and have to hide your true personality then you're not truly free. At some point you're going to resent your partner, even though it probably isn't your partner's fault in any way. And, of course, it works in reverse. If you're very uptight and can't accept your partner's true personality then your partner can't be free in your presence.

So let's take a look at some taboos and how, if they're your taboos, you might break them.

TALKING DIRTY

Possibly there are sex words that are taboo as far as you're concerned. You would never normally use them. During sex, however, different standards can apply and the same words that had seemed offensive can be very exciting and even liberating.

Breaking the taboo
Next time you're having sex, rather than use euphemisms for parts of the body, use the 'dirty' words and see what effect they have.

SEXUAL FANTASIES

Just about everyone has sexual fantasies. There's no reason at all to feel guilty or ashamed about that. A fantasy could be imagining something quite commonplace you'd like to do with your current partner, but never have. Or it could be something rather exotic, such as being forced to take part in an orgy. Men and women tend to have only slightly different fantasy lives. The main difference is that men's fantasies are usually more active and more explicit with plenty of 'close-ups'.

The kinds of things men like to fantasize about are:

▶ *sex with their current partners*
▶ *oral sex*
▶ *sex with two women*
▶ *being especially dominant*
▶ *being submissive*
▶ *reliving past sexual encounters*
▶ *watching.*

The kinds of things women like to fantasize about are:

▶ *sex with their current partners*
▶ *new techniques*
▶ *sex in romantic places*
▶ *being watched undressing, masturbating or making love*
▶ *being found irresistible*
▶ *being forced to have sex*
▶ *sex with a close woman friend*
▶ *sex with a celebrity.*

Breaking the taboo
Agreeing to exchange sexual fantasies can certainly be both surprising and mind-expanding because you'll discover things about your partner you probably never imagined.

A good time is during sex itself. Float your least threatening idea and see what happens. If you're worried about it, you could dress it up as something you dreamed. For example, you could say:

▶ *'Last night I dreamed people were watching us while we made love.'*

- ▶ 'Last night I dreamed another woman was in a changing room with me.'
- ▶ 'Last night I dreamed I was your sex slave.'

If you sense your partner freeze up then say no more. But it doesn't necessarily mean your partner isn't interested. He or she may simply need time to reflect on this development. Or it may be that you chose the wrong kind of fantasy. Hopefully, though, your partner will have responded either by taking the fantasy further, or by introducing a new fantasy in which case your sex life now has a whole new dimension.

Sometimes it happens that the person who first opened the door to fantasies is shocked by the response. If your partner reveals things you weren't expecting, reflect that fantasies don't necessarily indicate real-life desires.

Insight

In order to be able to handle your partner's sexual fantasies, you must sweep aside double standards and hypocrisy. Reflect honestly on your own fantasies and don't be judgemental. But both of you will need to proceed cautiously. Being able to recount all of your sexual fantasies, and to handle all of your partner's, is an ideal but it's one you may never attain.

MASTURBATION

Just as most men and women fantasize, so most men and women masturbate. If your masturbation is a secret from your partner, then neither of you is truly free. As a general rule, men masturbate more when they're *not* having enough sex with their partners, while women masturbate more when they *are* having enough sex with their partners. But, essentially, solo masturbation isn't a comment on your relationship because it's simply a completely different thing to lovemaking.

Breaking the taboo

In Tantric sex, women are goddesses and openly display their *yonis*, which traditionally were seen as a source of magic.

Sit comfortably on your bed, lean back against some pillows, open your legs and unashamedly display your *yoni* to your partner. Some Tantric texts refer to the *yoni* being ringed with hair but most men seem to find a clear view the most exciting. Then play with yourself however you normally do.

Women are not usually anywhere near as excited by the sight of a man's *lingam* as a man is by the sight of a woman's *yoni*. But there's a very good reason why a man should feel absolutely free not only to display his erect *lingam* but to play with it in front of his partner. The fact is that when an erection goes down, the surest way for a man to be able to get it back again is to masturbate. When a man *knows* he can self-stimulate in front of his partner without any embarrassment whatsoever, he's less likely to have problems in the first place (anxiety is the enemy of erection) and more likely to be able to get his erection back quickly.

It can be nice to have a masturbation session together, either lying side by side or sitting opposite one another.

Showing your partner how you masturbate is a good way of demonstrating how you like your body to be pleasured. Be completely open about what you like to do to yourself.

ANAL STIMULATION

Tantrikas don't categorize parts of the body as 'good' or 'bad'. But many non-Tantrikas do, and for them nothing is more 'bad' than the anus. Yet in men, the anus is second only to the penis as a potential source of pleasure. In women it's second to the clitoris and approximately on a par with the vagina (some women rate it more highly, some less). So breaking the taboo about the anus is well worth doing.

Breaking the taboo
▸ **Step 1:** *Excite yourself in your normal way then explore your anus with a lubricated finger. Run it round and round the outside. If that feels nice, push your finger (nail well trimmed)*

inside a little way. Explore the sensations you can create.
See what feels good and what doesn't.

▶ **Step 2:** *Have sex in your normal way and when excitement*
has built up place a lubricated finger on your partner's anus
and use a circling motion. If your partner responds you can go
further by gently pushing your finger (nail well trimmed) in a
little way. Ask if it feels nice. Ask what you can do to make it
feel even better.

▶ **Step 3:** *Tell your partner exactly how you like your own anus*
to be stimulated.

There's a great deal more to anal stimulation which is why it gets a
section to itself (see Chapter 9).

SEX OUT OF DOORS

Kaula ceremonies were generally under the stars. On nights
dictated by the moon, the participants would gather either in a
relatively remote location, such as the top of a hill, or in a place
others were unlikely to go in the dark, such as a cremation
ground.

For the aristocracy, however, such locations were a little too rough
and, around the end of the first millennium, the wealthy began
to commission permanent roofless enclosures (so the semi-divine
yoginis we met in Chapter 1 could descend from the sky into the
bodies of the women to have sex with the waiting men). Known
as sixty-four-*yogini* temples, they had 64 (or sometimes 60) stone
images of *yoginis* in niches around the stone perimeter and a Shiva
icon in the middle.

Breaking the taboo
Before contemplating sex out of doors yourself make sure you
know the law. In some countries, including Britain, sex out
of doors is not an offence as long as you have a reasonable
expectation that no one can see you. In other countries the
penalties can be severe. But let's assume there's no legal problem
where you are.

Without a nice comfortable bed, sex out of doors can seem second best, but making love under the stars or in a beautiful natural setting on a warm, sunny day can be wonderful, consciousness-expanding experiences. You'll certainly feel much closer to solving the secret of the universe. When the terrain offers no help, the easiest position is *yab yum*. All you, the man, have to do is sit cross-legged on the ground. You, the woman, then sit on your partner's lap, facing him. If the ground is hard, some clothes will make a cushion. (For full details of this and other 'outdoor' positions see Chapter 10.)

EROTICA

If erotica is a taboo with one or both of you, then it's a taboo you should consider breaking. Yes, there are certain kinds of pornography that no right-minded person should have anything to do with, but there's also erotica that's arousing, beautiful and instructive. And mind-expanding in the sense of giving you new ideas.

If you're a man, you probably watch erotica on DVD or the internet and if your partner doesn't know, then that's the first thing to tackle. Tell her and be freed from the furtive life. Invite her to watch something with you.

If you're a woman, you're far more likely to say that erotic films are boring, and to believe it. But the scientific evidence, in terms of vaginal wetness and other measures, is that women get far more aroused than they admit, or realize. It also depends very much on attitude. Erotica *is* boring if you just sit and watch. The whole idea is to join in. Just as if, in fact, you were taking part in the *cakrapuja*.

Breaking the taboo
▶ **Step 1:** *Some time before you intend to have Tantric sex, one or both of you should review snippets of the erotica to make sure it doesn't go too far for you.*

- ▶ **Step 2:** *Get ready for your Tantric sex session as described in this book and, once you're in the mood, begin to watch.*
- ▶ **Step 3:** *Make love using the erotica as a background, just as if you and the actors were together in the* cakrapuja.

Warning: A danger of erotica is that the man tries to force his partner to copy things against her will. That is not acceptable. Erotica should be a source of inspiration, not coercion.

THE SEX SHOP

Although there are sex shops in most towns, they're still a taboo for many people. To overcome this resistance, many dress their windows with lingerie and keep the sex toys at the back.

Breaking the taboo

Try to go together as a couple. You'll probably see things you'd like to buy but don't feel quite ready to admit to. That's ok; you can always come back another time. There's no hurry. But make up your minds that, whatever happens, you will buy *something*. Some women like to go as a group and have a good laugh but, be warned, you'll need a lot of courage to buy anything in front of your friends. If there's no convenient sex shop or you're too embarrassed to go in, then take a look at the internet shopping suggestions in Taking it further.

TALKING ABOUT SEX

Talking about sex is an amazingly prevalent taboo and one that takes a very long time to overcome fully. Some people are simply embarrassed while others think talking will somehow destroy the magic. Believe me, the opposite is the case. The truth is that talking about sex is mind-expanding. In my focus groups I often find that someone will take the opportunity to reveal something they'd always wanted to say, to the absolute astonishment of their partner. No doubt they go home and have very good sex afterwards.

Breaking the taboo
- ▶ **Step 1:** *If you're not used to talking about sex, you have to find some way of getting started. Since you're reading this book, an obvious way is to ask your partner if she or he agrees with something I've written. (If your partner doesn't know you're reading it, try leaving it somewhere obvious.) You might also take advantage of a TV programme or a film to discuss an issue that's been raised.*
- ▶ **Step 2:** *Once you've opened the way to talking about sex, never risk closing it down by saying anything critical. Always look for a positive way to express your feelings. For example, don't say, 'You're too rough with my clitoris.' Instead, say, 'When you tickle my clitoris ever so gently it drives me absolutely wild.'*
- ▶ **Step 3:** *Gradually, over the weeks, work your way towards the issues that are the most personal and profound.*

Liberation from the cycle of death and rebirth is one of the aims of Tantric sex. Learning to talk about your sexual desires frankly and without embarrassment is a form of liberation in itself.

DEATH

Death is the ultimate taboo. No one wants to talk about it and no one wants to die. But some Tantrikas deliberately chose to confront death by having sex at cremation grounds. And those were not nice tidy places like a modern crematorium. There would have been bones and bits of unburned body lying around and scavenged upon by wild animals. At night they would have been terrifying places. The following supplication gives a flavour of the kind of thing that went on:

> *O Goddess Kali, he who on a Tuesday midnight having uttered your mantra, makes an offering to you in the cremation ground just once of a [pubic] hair from his female partner pulled out by the root, wet with semen poured from*

his penis into her menstruating vagina, becomes a great poet,
a Lord of the World, and always travels on elephant-back.

From the *Karpuradistotra*, Sri Mahakala

As bizarre as it sounds, there was a logic to it all. The point is
that there's an enormous difference between believing something
you've been taught and actually experiencing it for yourself. This
kind of Tantric sex was all about trying to have that experience.
We all know, for example, that we must die. And yet we don't
really know it. That's to say, we don't live our lives as we logically
should. We don't, if Hindus, always live like people who will
be reincarnated in accordance with our conduct in this life. We
don't, if Christians, always turn the other cheek or accept that
the wealthy can't go to Heaven. And few of us live with any
intensity. The seers of Tantrism reasoned that it needed something
as extreme and dramatic as sex at a cremation ground to truly
confront the reality of death. And some Western poets have
followed the same line of thought, as in these lines by Andrew
Marvell (1621–78):

But at my back I always hear
Time's wingéd chariot hurrying near...
The grave's a fine and private place,
But none I think do there embrace...

Breaking the taboo
You probably don't want to have sex in a cemetery and you might
get arrested if you try, but there are other things you could do
to confront yourself with the reality of death. Certainly visit a
graveyard and reflect on the shortness of life. If you are a religious
person, look again at your sacred texts and pay attention to what
they have to say. Maybe volunteer to work in an old people's
home; it could help you and it'll certainly help them. Above all,
make the most of every day, every hour and every minute – which
means having plenty of Tantric sex.

10 THINGS TO REMEMBER

1 *Breaking taboos and overcoming inhibitions are important aspects of Tantric sex.*

2 *No one should use Tantric sex as an excuse to try to force a partner into things they don't want to do.*

3 *The most common taboos to be broken among Hindu followers of Tantra were the prohibition on meat, fish, alcohol and group sex, but you can elect to tackle your own personal taboos.*

4 *Large quantities of alcohol are the enemy of good sex but sharing a small quantity from a 'ceremonial container' can help create the right atmosphere, while a little drink after sex will prolong the dopamine 'hit'.*

5 *The* cakrapuja *(group sex) was at the heart of the* Kaula *Tantric rites, but you can adapt almost all the techniques for the privacy of your own bedroom.*

6 *Being uninhibited doesn't mean doing things you don't want to do, but doing things you do want to do but have been afraid of.*

7 *Sharing your sexual fantasies can be a powerful way of expanding your minds by learning more about one another, while 'talking dirty' can increase sexual excitement.*

8 *You should be free to masturbate in front of one another.*

9 *Breaking the taboo over anal stimulation opens up an entirely new erogenous frontier.*

10 *Sex out of doors (where legal) can bring about a sense of oneness with nature and at night, under the stars, with the whole cosmos.*

HOW TANTRIC ARE YOU NOW?

- ☐ Have you made up your mind to rid yourself of inhibitions?
- ☐ Have you broken any personal taboos to arouse your partner?
- ☐ Have you tried a little alcohol *after* sex, to prolong your dopamine 'hit' (while keeping your alcohol consumption *down* before sex)?
- ☐ Have you tried 'talking dirty' during sex?
- ☐ Have you told your partner any of your sexual fantasies?
- ☐ Have you been able to hear your partner's sexual fantasies without being judgemental?
- ☐ Have you masturbated in front of your partner?
- ☐ Have you happily encouraged your partner to masturbate in front of you?
- ☐ Have you tried stimulating your anus or encouraged your partner to stimulate it?
- ☐ Have you tried stimulating your partner's anus?
- ☐ Have you tried erotica?
- ☐ Have you had sex out of doors?

If you answered 'yes' to between nine and twelve questions you obviously don't have very many taboos and are fully open to expanding your consciousness through sex.

If you answered 'yes' to between six and eight questions you're on your way but you have quite a bit of experimenting to do.

If you couldn't answer 'yes' to more than five questions, you're allowing too many taboos to get in the way of your sex life and the development of your mind – read the chapter again and really work on breaking taboos that have no real justification.

4

....

Mantra – the Tantric vibrator

In this chapter you will learn:
* *how mantras were the original vibrators*
* *how to choose and use modern vibrators*
* *how to use* pranayama *to control sexual arousal.*

> *He does not touch a yantra nor make japa of mantra at*
> *night... He regards a mantra as being merely letters only.*
> *Such a one is called pashu, and he is the worst kind of man.*
>
> Kubjika Tantra

If you've ever bought any kind of sex toy, then you've probably
bought a vibrator. If you did, you're probably having a wonderful
time with it. And, when you think about it, that's really rather
curious, because men and women don't normally stimulate
themselves or one another with vibrations. They caress, stroke,
lick, thrust, circle and so on, but they don't vibrate.

Or do they?

Probably no insight into the nature of the universe is as impressive
as the perception in Tantra (and some other Eastern beliefs and
religions) that the universe is essentially composed of nothing more
(or less) than vibrations. And that includes you and your partner.
Many hundreds of years after those ancient mystics first made their
discovery, this theory has now been confirmed by Western science.
We now know that atoms are not solid building blocks but systems

of particles that circulate or vibrate at fantastic speeds. Which effectively means that you and I aren't as solid as we thought (see the factbox below). And it may explain why vibrators have such a powerful effect.

The Tantric mystics didn't have microscopes and telescopes and all the rest of the scientific instruments we have today. So how did they work these things out? According to the *Upanishads*, the Hindu spiritual treatises, the reality of the universe can only be grasped during a state of consciousness that is different to normal consciousness, a consciousness of joy. In other words, during sex. Now I can't prove they intuited these ideas during lengthy Tantric sex sessions but I like to think so. It's during those moments of radiant ecstasy that we can apprehend things beyond the capabilities of our normal senses. As the followers of *Tantra* say: 'Spirit can alone know Spirit.'

Of course, the early Tantrikas didn't have little electric motors to produce sexual vibrations. But they did have other ways of producing vibrations. They had bells and drums and gongs and, most of all, mantras.

The vibrating universe

At school you may have been taught that everything was composed of tiny atoms. A teacher did a drawing on a blackboard of a large circle representing the hard exterior of the atom with a small solid circle in the middle, representing the nucleus. But if an atom were to be magnified to the size of the dome of St Paul's Cathedral in London, the nucleus would still only be the size of a grain of salt and the other subatomic particles would be like a few specks of dust. What's more, none of those particles are ever still. The protons and neutrons in the nucleus zoom around at 40,000 miles per second while the electrons circle at about 600 miles a second. Thus a human being is mostly empty

(Contd)

space in which tiny particles rocket about at mind-boggling speeds. You are mostly empty space. And, as empty space, it's really just an artificial construction to see yourself as something separate from your partner and from the rest of the mostly empty space that is the universe. (*Maya*, which conceals the true reality, is at work.) If that wasn't already amazing enough, reflect on this. The atoms of which you at this very moment are composed will have been part of several stars and literally millions of Earthly organisms before becoming part of you. In all probability, some of the atoms of which you are at this moment composed previously made up Confucius, **Buddha**, and any other historical figure you care to mention. I say 'at this moment' because your atoms are constantly being recycled. Today, you are not the same person you were last month. In which case, who or what is the real you?

This constant change is all part of Tantra's 'cosmic dance', with everything in continual motion. In fact, as you're reading this, cosmic rays are passing right through you. Fortunately, you won't feel a thing and this process of constant creation and destruction even applies to the entire universe itself. One day, Hindus believe, it will contract to a dot, only to begin all over again with another Big Bang. They believe this cycle will repeat itself again and again. Some modern scientists agree, and some disagree.

Getting in the mood with mantras

A mantra spoken out loud is a mixture of vibration, breath and meaning. It isn't a prayer because the meaning of a prayer is entirely in the words whereas the meaning of a mantra, while it may be partially in the word or words, is also in the sound. It isn't enough merely to mutter a mantra or to speak it without knowledge. Mantras have to be intoned in the proper way, according to *svara* (rhythm) and *varna* (intonation). Tantrikas believe they are then extremely powerful because they, as it were, resonate with the divine vibration of the cosmos.

Have a go
We'll have a look at mantras in a little more detail in a moment, but let's have a little fun with sounds right now, in a way not originally intended.

▶ **Step 1:** *Put your mouth on some particularly sensitive part of your partner's body. The penis, clitoris, and the entire vulva are the most obvious places to try this out, but the neck is also pretty good.*
▶ **Step 2:** *Choose any short word ending in 'm' and intone it.*
▶ **Step 3:** *Keep that 'm' humming as long as possible. Your aim is to make the flesh vibrate – just in the same way, in fact, that a vibrator would.*
▶ **Step 4:** *Ask your partner for feedback, varying the sound and the pressure until you get an exciting effect.*

The role of the guru

According to Tantric thought, when it comes to your personal mantra, you can't just choose anything you like. Your personal mantra should be bestowed on you by a guru who has got to know you and given the matter careful thought. Your guru will have learned mantras from his or her guru, who in turn learned them from another guru, and so on back through the ages.

And there are other reasons for seeking a guru. The guru combines the role of yogi (mainly concerned with enjoyment or *bhoga*) and that of *jnani*, a knowledgeable person concerned with *moksha* (liberation). As it says in the tenth century *Tantraloka*, 'he who wishes enjoyment, liberation and knowledge, should seek out a guru who is well-practised...'

And that's exactly the problem. The chances of finding a genuine guru, let alone being accepted as a *shishya* (see the factbox below) are exceedingly small.

Finding a guru

Ideally, a guru wouldn't be found by looking in any kind of directory. You should go to India and wander. They say that when the moment is right the guru appears. They also say that only the person who is fit for a teacher is able to recognize him or her.

But in the rest of the world you might never encounter a guru by chance so take a look at Taking it further. Given that there are so many different kinds of Tantra, make sure your guru teaches the style you want.

If you become a disciple you'll be a *shishya* and your relationship with your guru will continue until *siddhi* or success. Another word for you, as we've seen, would be a *sadhaka*, which is someone who performs all the necessary *sadhanas* or rites.

The reason that only a guru can achieve special things is that, in fact, he or she is nothing other than the mouthpiece of the 'Supreme Guru' who, ultimately, is God. In other words, it's actually the Supreme Guru who is instructing you, through the voice of the earthly guru. That is why, in some sects, a guru is treated as a god.

OM

If you can't find a guru to select a mantra and teach you *svara* and *varna* what should you do? Well, let's see if I can teach you, through the written word, how to intone the most famous mantra of all, *OM*.

Tantrikas believe that:

▶ OM *is the sound – the vibration – of cosmic energy in its pure state*
▶ OM *created galaxies*
▶ OM *is the* **bija** *or seed-syllable of the universe*
▶ OM *brings humans into intuitive contact with, as it were, the secret of the universe.*

Have a go
▶ **Step 1:** *Begin by opening your mouth wide and, as if yawning, exhale an 'aah' sound (as when the doctor examines your throat).*
▶ **Step 2:** *Almost immediately narrow your mouth slightly into an 'O' shape, so the sound evolves from 'aah' to 'oh'.*
▶ **Step 3:** *Move your tongue to the back of your mouth to block the glottis and produce an 'ong' sound as in 'gong'. (In the previous exercise I told you to make an 'mmm' sound but that was just for fun to get your lips vibrating. To sound* OM *in the authentic way, the mouth must remain open throughout.)*
▶ **Step 4:** *Produce a group of* OMs *on one breath by releasing the tongue to produce the 'aah-oh' and then replacing it to create the 'ong'. The result is like a continuous 'ng' drone, punctuated by the 'aah-oh'.*
▶ **Step 5:** *Try to get the* OM *vibrations affecting as much of your body as you can, right down to the genitals if possible.*

So how does this fit in with Tantric sex? As you now know, Tantra is a spiritual path. Intoning *OM* is a kind of meditation. Some Tantrikas even focus exclusively on mantras as their spiritual path. They don't have sex. But you will. And by intoning *OM* beforehand, you remind yourself that Tantric sex is all about *ananda.* You can also intone *OM* during the special Tantric foreplay known as *nyasa* (see Chapter 5). But the silent style of mantra, which I'll deal with next, is probably the one you'll use the most.

Om mani padme Hum

After OM itself, the next most well-known mantra is probably the Buddhist *Om mani padme Hum*, which is usually translated as 'jewel in the lotus'. But the meaning is, in fact, sexual. *Mani* (jewel) is the Buddhist equivalent of the Hindu *vajra* (diamond) and both symbolize the *lingam*. In the light of that, you won't be surprised to learn that *padme* (lotus) stands for the *yoni*. The whole mantra is essentially saying the basis of the whole universe is the penis in the vagina – sex.

Internal mantras for sex

In a busy world it can sometimes be very difficult to get in the right frame of mind for Tantric sex. Nevertheless, the right frame of mind is essential if you're going to achieve *ananda*. Spending a few minutes meditating on an internal mantra is a great way of both slowing down and focusing your thoughts on the whole purpose of what you're going to be doing. The mantra I'm going to give you is *So Hum* which means 'I am Brahman' – Tantrikas reason that if Brahman created everything in the universe then anything in the universe is Brahman, including you.

If you find it difficult to accept that idea, then you could focus on the alternative translation, 'I am bliss'. Or you could devise your own, more practical, mantra. For example, to help control ejaculation, a man might inwardly repeat, 'Don't come.' (We'll be looking in detail at ejaculation control in Chapters 7 and 8.) Or you might find it helpful to repeat 'I'm relaxed' or 'I'm free' or, in a more Tantric vein, 'God…dess' or 'He's god'. It's up to you. Remember that we're only talking about *internal* mantras. Out loud, these kinds of phrases just wouldn't resonate correctly.

Repeating a mantra over and over is known as *japa* (and is the basis of Transcendental Meditation). If you've ever been on any courses in self-motivation or confidence you'll recognize at once the power of repetition.

Have a go
- ▶ Step 1: *Sit comfortably cross-legged on the floor, a couch, or the bed with your hands resting open, palms upwards, on your knees.*
- ▶ Step 2: *Breathe in quite naturally and as you do so 'say' So in your mind while moving the ring finger of your left hand to touch the base of your left thumb. (Keep your right hand still.)*
- ▶ Step 3: *Breathe out quite naturally and as you do so 'say' Hum in your mind while returning your ring finger to its starting point. (If you choose another mantra, you'll need to split it into two parts in just the same way, to synchronize with the movement of your finger.)*
- ▶ Step 4: *Once you've established a rhythm, close your eyes and continue like this for a few minutes while inwardly also visualizing the movement of your finger.*

The ring finger of your left hand is related to the *Anahata* chakra (see Chapter 2) while the pad at the base of the thumb is known as 'Shukra's mount' or the 'mount of Venus'. When you unite the two you are symbolically opening your heart to love through sex. Be sure not to force the breathing as you do it. Just be natural. The co-ordination and visualization skills should keep your mind free of other thoughts. However, if thoughts do come into your mind just let them pass.

Be noisy sometimes

The Tantras say that there is also what might be called 'informal mantras'. According to Abhinavagupta in the *Tantraloka*, a mantra can be the 'unvoiced syllable' which bursts from 'the throat of a beautiful woman, in the form of an unintentional sound, without forethought or concentration.' *Ha-ha* is such a mantra, according to Jayaratha's commentary to the *Tantraloka*, denoting that a woman is 'savouring everlasting bliss'.

In my focus groups I'm always surprised by the number of people who have sex without speaking or, apparently, making much noise. The psychoanalyst Wilhelm Reich, who was a disciple of Freud, wrote quite confidently in his *Die Funktion des Orgasmus* (The Function of the Orgasm, 1927) that:

> *With the exception of endearments, orgasmic men and women never laugh or talk during intercourse. Both talking and laughing suggest a serious inability to surrender oneself...*

While I hesitate to contradict such a famous specialist, my own view is that while there's a time to be quiet and contemplative in Tantric sex, there's also a time to be noisy. In the previous chapter I looked at the breaking of any taboos you might have about 'dirty' words and the telling of fantasies. Such words, and the phrases that evoke fantasies, can act as mantras along with all the wordless noises, the moans, groans, whimpers, shrieks, yells, whoops, howls, hums, growls and all the rest. Don't be afraid of them.

Have a go
- ▶ Step 1: *Begin to have sex without using either words or sounds.*
- ▶ Step 2: *After a few minutes, allow yourselves to make whatever noises you wish. Experiment with the full range from little whimpers up to screams and yells. Don't hold anything back.*
- ▶ Step 3: *Introduce whatever words or phrases come into your heads. They could be romantic ('I love you'), they could be spiritual ('You are the goddess') or they could be entirely erotic ('You are so dirty'). Don't be inhibited.*
- ▶ Step 4: *Repeat Steps 1 to 3.*
- ▶ Step 5: *After sex, discuss the different effects.*

Artificial vibrators

As we've seen, mantras can act as vibrators of the body. But, nowadays, we have special vibrators for sex. Would the original Tantrikas have used them? I'm sure they would. A *vira*, that's to say a guru of 'heroic status' might have had sex with up to 108 women in a single session and to do that he might well have used a dildo, or as the *Kama Sutra* called it, an *apadravya* (although it would also have been possible using the techniques of semen retention described in Chapter 8). So these kinds of devices go almost as far back as the invention of sex.

STANDARD VIBRATORS

The most popular sex toy is the vibrator and they do things that human beings just can't manage. Once you've been on the end of one, especially if you're a woman, you'll never want to exclude them from your sexual repertoire. A man can rub his finger backwards and forwards on his partner's clitoris several times a second but that's nowhere near as fast as a vibrator. Quite apart from which, it's just not something a man can keep up for very long whereas a vibrator can continue indefinitely. A vibrator, then, is an essential piece of equipment for any woman who doesn't orgasm easily.

The most popular vibrator models are designed to look like a *lingam*. Some are extremely realistic while others merely approximate the general shape and size. Inside there's a little motor, powered by batteries, that sets up a vibration. Although it's quite different to the kind of stimulation provided by 'normal' sex, it's nevertheless highly effective. Some vibrators are made of a fairly soft plastic, which seems less intimidating, but the hard plastic models transmit the vibrations better. To be frank, quite a lot of them do look rather tacky which is where the new glass models come in (see p. 80).

It's easy to see what the woman can get out of a vibrator, but what about the man? Well, for a start, the Tantric style of sex is all about sharing joy. If the woman is happy the man should be happy too. But, as we'll see, there are some direct benefits for a man.

How do you use it? At first, most men will probably want to take charge of the vibrator. Well, that's just how men are. If it's anything mechanical they simply assume that only they will be able to understand it. But, in reality, it's much better if the woman uses it on herself. For a start, although most vibrators are designed to look like penises, they're not at their best when they're thrust in and out of the vagina. They're far more effective when they're held still on or beside the clitoris, depending on sensitivity. That's why it's best to leave a woman to do it to herself, because only she knows exactly the optimum part of her anatomy to hold it against. While that's going on, a man can be simply watching, which is already quite good fun, or he could be holding his lover in his arms and feeling her orgasm. Or he could be inside her in which case he might feel the vibrations as well. Alternatively, he could be using his own vibrator. Held against the shaft of the penis or the glans a vibrator can induce some very enjoyable sensations in a man. Or it can be stroked against the perineum and anal area.

Have a go – exploring vibrators
Make sure that the packaging on your vibrator hasn't been disturbed. Unwrap it and, if it's the plastic battery-powered kind, wash it with soap and water, taking care that no water gets into the battery compartment. Wash again after each use. If it's a mains-powered model, follow the hygiene instructions that come with it.

FOR A MAN ON A WOMAN
The first rule is communication. Keep checking with your partner how she's feeling and whether she wants more pressure or less pressure and so on.

Although the vibrator is probably shaped like a penis, don't immediately begin thrusting it in and out. Take time to explore your partner's body and let her experience the new sensations it can create. First of all, raise the level of excitement a little by using the vibrator near her clitoris. If your partner is very sensitive in this area begin on a slow speed and apply it against her underwear. Gradually increase the intensity by turning up the speed, applying to bare skin and moving in steps closer and closer to the clitoris. Don't constantly move the vibrator around; rather move it ½ cm (or ¼″) at a time and hold it in the new position for a while.

Once you've woken her body up, try the vibrator in different places. Circle her breasts with it, then her areolae, then her nipples. A vibrator can also do interesting things in the small of the neck and on the feet.

Now put some lubricant on the vibrator and on the entrance to her vagina. This is very important. Gently introduce the vibrator 5 cm (2″). As she relaxes into the sensations so you can slide it a little further. Remember that a *yoni* is only as long as a finger so, whatever you do, don't attempt to thrust the whole length of the vibrator into her; that will only cause pain. Now try sliding the vibrator backwards and forwards with short movements. In all probability she won't find this particularly enjoyable but she may and it's all part of experimenting to see what feels good. Also try pressing the vibrator against her **G-spot** – in other words, apply a little pressure in the direction of her pubic mound. Some vibrators are curved to make this easier to do. Finally, return to her vulva and gently hold the vibrator as close as she wants to her clitoris and keep it there, quite still, until she has an orgasm (Be ready to take it away as the orgasm ends because, at that point, it may cause pain.).

FOR A WOMAN ON HERSELF
In truth, it's usually better for a woman to use a vibrator on herself. She knows exactly what feels good and what doesn't and can handle the vibrator with precision.

When you're on your own the inclination is to go straight for the clitoris, but it's worth taking the time to explore the effect of the vibrator all over your body. Try the same things that I've suggested a man does.

Quite a lot of women instinctively react against putting anything unusual into their vaginas. If that includes you, try to overcome your resistance and explore the sensations the vibrator can create there. Use plenty of lubrication. You might enjoy having the vibrator in your vagina while at the same time stimulating your clitoris with your fingers. (And there are vibrators designed to stimulate the vagina and the clitoris simultaneously.) Also apply pressure so the vibrator works on the G-spot. But in all probability you'll find you want to hold the vibrator on or close to your clitoris, which is the surest way for most women to orgasm.

FOR A WOMAN ON A MAN
When you're making love with your partner and using a vibrator on yourself, there's no reason you shouldn't also use it on him. Try it on his nipples and on different places on the shaft of his penis as well as the glans.

FOR A MAN ON HIMSELF
Try holding the vibrator against different places on your penis. You'll find it can bring you to orgasm. You could also buy an artificial vagina which has been designed more precisely for male pleasure.

DURING INTERCOURSE
During intercourse, try holding the vibrator against the base of the penis. That way, both of you should feel the sensations. When a woman is lying face down on the bed, another good way of using a vibrator is to slide it underneath against the vulva.

GLASS DILDOS AND VIBRATORS

In the last few years we've seen the appearance of glass dildos (false *lingams* but without the vibrations) in all kinds of beautiful shapes, often with strands of different colours embedded within them. Some of them are so elegant they actually look like pieces of art. If one of your children or your grandmother spots yours you can always explain it away as a bedside sculpture.

Why would anybody want a dildo, a *Kama Sutra* style *apadravya*, when modern technology has improved the concept with a motor? The answer is that a lot of these dildos are designed specifically for the G-spot. As we'll see in Chapter 7, the G-spot is that slightly rougher area on the roof of the vagina just inside the entrance. A good dildo is designed to hit it every time and, in fact, it's not necessary to have vibrations for the G-spot because it seems to respond best to simple pressure. Choose a design with a chunky rounded head for the most effective stimulation. Certainly a dildo can be thrust in and out, but the most effective thing is to insert it and then use the PC muscle to squeeze it against the G-spot (refer back to Chapter 2 if you've forgotten about the PC). However if you do want vibrations, you can either set your dildo alive by touching a conventional vibrator to the base or, in some cases, buy a special vibrating device that fits into a hole in the dildo.

Apart from the fact that glass dildos look and feel so much nicer than plastic ones they have the advantage of being unbreakable. Well, almost. In fact, they're usually made from pyrex which means you can even put them in the dishwasher. (That may take some explaining if your dinner guests insist on loading the dishwasher for you!) Pyrex has some other advantages over plastic. You can stand your dildo in warm water so it matches your body temperature or, for a completely different sensation, you can put it in the fridge for a while. Another point about glass is that, being so smooth, it doesn't need any artificial lubricant. Or, at any rate very little.

SPECIALIST VIBRATORS

Humans being the incredibly inventive creatures that they are, it shouldn't come as any surprise that the basic vibrator has been improved in all sorts of ways. Fortunately, they're not very expensive so, over a period of time, you can experiment with different designs:

▶ **Mains powered models.** *Any woman who really has difficulty achieving orgasm, even with a battery-powered vibrator,* *should consider a mains-powered model. There are two basic sorts. One style doubles as a massager, a very nice idea because it means you can both use it all over your bodies. The other is more specifically designed for use on the clitoris and inside the vagina. Women who orgasm easily should use these very powerful models with caution because they can quickly take you beyond pleasure into a state of numbness.*

▶ **Clitoral vibrators.** *Women like plenty of clitoral stimulation so the designers have come up with two different solutions. One is to add some sort of vibrating nub to a conventional vibrator. The most famous is the 'rabbit' whose latex ears tickle the clitoris while the main barrel is inside the vagina. The other style does away with vaginal stimulation altogether and just concentrates on the vulva. Some of these look like showerheads with a stippled pad to arouse the inner labia as well as the clitoris.*

▶ **Fingertip vibrators.** *These slip onto a finger so wherever you touch your partner you create an electrifying effect.*

▶ **Nipple vibrators.** *If you're easily aroused by nipple stimulation these vibrating clamps will excite you very quickly; if not, man or woman, they can 'teach' your nipples to become more responsive.*

▶ **Novelty vibrators.** *There are remote-controlled vibrators, vibrators that respond when your mobile rings, vibrators built into inflatable cushions that you use like space hoppers, vibrators that keep time to music... If you've thought of it, somebody has probably made it.*

SPECIFICALLY FOR MEN

It's a fact that most sex toys are designed for women, but there are two kinds of sex toys for men that are particularly useful for Tantric sex. A third kind, for stimulating the prostate gland, is dealt with below under Anal toys.

Vibrating cock rings
If you have a problem maintaining an erection throughout lengthy Tantric sex sessions a vibrating cock ring could be the answer.

The old-fashioned cock rings that were designed to keep the *lingam* hard by constricting the outward flow of blood risked doing damage. This new generation of rings doesn't constrict the penis but work by maintaining constant stimulation.

The first were cumbersome affairs with wires leading to a battery pack but the latest designs are extremely light, don't have wires and are powered by built-in watch batteries.

Of course, it's not just the man who feels the pleasure. There's usually a little raised nub to work on the clitoris and, at the same time, the vibrations are transmitted along the penis and can therefore be felt inside the vagina.

Vibrating *yonis*

These are designed for men to use on their own or, perhaps, while their partners are masturbating with a vibrator. Because of the very realistic feel and intense stimulation, they make an excellent training device for practising the 'lock' and all the other techniques for controlling ejaculation that you'll be learning in Chapters 7 and 8.

Insight

Even if you've overcome any reservations about standard vibrators, you may still have doubts about anal sex and anal toys. To many people the whole subject sounds 'dirty' in every sense. But, in Tantric sex, everything is holy, including the anus. We'll be looking at the subject in detail in Chapter 9.

Yantra – the erotic abstract

A *yantra* in its most general sense is any instrument by which something is accomplished. Here we're concerned with *yantras* as sort of abstract designs. I say 'sort of' because although they may look a little like Western abstract art, they're not really abstract at all but energy diagrams with specific meanings. So, in a way, they're visual mantras. They're usually rather intricate and geometric, with motifs repeated and with a central point (usually a dot or a *yoni*) on which worshippers can focus for meditation. The funny thing about *yantras* is that even as Westerners with no knowledge of Tantra we can look at them and somehow feel that they're 'right'. On some level, they still speak to us.

In *puja*, a *yantra* is worshipped in the same way as any more obvious image. The *sadhaka* meditates upon a god, arouses the god within, and then communicates the divine presence to the *yantra* which he or she then worships. *Yantras* can also be used to improve concentration. And they can be used, as I'll be doing in a moment, in a sexual way.

Have a go – traditional method
▶ Step 1: *Find your* yantra *in a book of Tantric art, or online.*
▶ Step 2: *Place your* yantra *where you can easily see it. Begin by taking in the whole design. Just let your eyes roam back and forth, taking in the various elements.*
▶ Step 3: *Gradually let your focus be drawn in to the centre where there will be a small circle or dot or* yoni *symbol. Concentrate on that. Don't stare and don't glaze over; just look. Don't fight thoughts that come and go but always bring your attention back to the centre afterwards. (One benefit of the exercise is learning to focus on just one thing for a long time.)*
▶ Step 4: *Close your eyes and try to 'see' the image.*
▶ Step 5: *Gradually lengthen the sessions.*

Have a go – Western method
▶ Step 1: *Create your own* yantra *by taking a photograph of your partner's* yoni *or* lingam *(a digital image that you can view on your computer is best). Compose the shot so that there's a central point to focus on (such as the opening of the* yoni*).*
▶ Step 2: *Meditate for a little while on your partner as a goddess or god.*
▶ Step 3: *Now look at the* yantra, *which is the* yoni *or* lingam *of the goddess or god who is your partner.*

▶ **Step 4:** *After having let your eyes roam all over the image, focus on the central point. Concentrate on that. Don't stare and don't glaze over; just look. Keep thinking how this is the* yoni *or* lingam *of a goddess or god with whom you'll be having sex and thereby entering into a more spiritual state of consciousness.*

▶ **Step 5:** *Close your eyes and try to 'see' the image.*

▶ **Step 6:** *Call up the image whenever you wish.*

Pranayama – the transcendent breath

As you may already have discovered, one of the effects of intoning mantras out loud is to alter your normal pattern of breathing and, with it, your state of mind. Now we're going to take the art of breathing a little bit further.

Most people give very little thought to the subject. After all, breathing happens automatically, with the body taking as much or as little oxygen as it needs. So why even think about manual control?

The reality is that breathing is about a lot more than taking in oxygen and getting rid of carbon dioxide. According to the *Swara Tantra*, a man should inhale the breath of his partner from her left nostril into his right nostril, savouring its scent and contemplating its potency. If he does this three hours after midnight, she (that is, Shakti, acting through her) will then bestow magical powers on him. In Tantra, the left nostril is *ida*, the *nadi* (channel) that carries cool 'moon' energy, while the right nostril is *pingala*, the *nadi* carrying hot 'sun' energy. I don't believe in magic, but it's certainly an intimate act that adds to the sense of shared experience and oneness.

What I do believe in is *pranayama*. *Pranayama* is usually said to be derived from *prana* (breath) and *yama* (control) but I'm persuaded by those who argue it's not *yama* but *ayama* meaning expansion. *Prana* also means 'vital energy' or 'life force', so in my view we're really talking about increasing the life force. When you do it together you're increasing the sexual energy that you're exchanging.

Have a go

▶ **Step 1:** *To make it easy to hear one another breathing, have sex in the* yab yum *position (Shiva sitting cross-legged with Shakti on his lap – see Chapter 10).*

▶ **Step 2:** *With* lingam *and* yoni *united, deliberately make short, rapid breaths; the* rechak *(exhalation) should be through your mouth with little moans or groans. Notice that you become more excited.*

▶ **Step 3:** *Switch to long, steady breaths with the* rechak *significantly longer than the* puraka *(inhalation) and with a short period of* kumbhaka *(retention) in between. Notice that you feel more in control (see Chapter 8 for further details on withholding ejaculation by* pranayama*).*

▶ **Step 4:** *Synchronize deep, rapid breaths. Let your stomachs swell with the* puraka *and pull your stomachs forcefully back towards your spines for the* rechak*. There should be no* kumbhaka*. Continue for not more than five minutes but stop sooner if you become seriously dizzy.*

▶ **Step 5:** *Assuming that you're not too dizzy, co-ordinate deep, rapid breathing so one person's* rechak *coincides with the other's* puraka*. Reflect on the fact that you're taking in air that has been inside your partner's body. Continue for up to another five minutes but, as before, stop if you become seriously dizzy.*

▶ **Step 6:** *Resume normal breathing and continue having sex.*

Once you've finished your experiments in *pranayama* discuss the effects. You should find that rapid breathing excites while steady breathing calms. Hyperventilation will accentuate some of the effects of sex, by making your body tingle and your brain a little dizzy – yogis believe that all great experiences take place in a condition of dizziness.

Hyperventilation

When you breathe faster and deeper than necessary (hyperventilation), you not only flush out carbon dioxide but reduce the level of carbonic acid in the blood (the form in which carbon dioxide is carried). That in turn means the blood becomes less acid. When the blood is less acid (more alkaline) the blood vessels constrict and the level of available calcium is reduced, causing tingling. Contrary to what many people imagine, deep breathing does not bathe the brain in more oxygen but the reverse because the cerebral vasoconstriction reduces the blood flow and leads to lightheadedness. In an extreme case a person might faint. Never overdo it.

10 THINGS TO REMEMBER

1 *The whole universe and everyone in it vibrates in the cosmic dance.*

2 *A* mantra *spoken out loud is a mixture of vibration, breath and meaning.*

3 *The chances of finding a genuine guru, let alone being accepted as a* shishya, *are exceedingly small, but this book can teach you a great deal.*

4 *Getting in the mood for Tantric sex means slowing down, which is something you can achieve by the use of a mantra.*

5 *The mantra* OM *is the sound – the vibration – of cosmic energy in its pure state.*

6 *The moans and groans made during sex can be 'informal mantras' – be uninhibited and let them out.*

7 *Buy a vibrator and experiment – the original Tantrikas would certainly have used them if they had been available.*

8 Yantras *are energy diagrams or 'visual mantras'.*

9 Pranayama *(energy expansion) can be used to increase or decrease excitement.*

10 *Hyperventilation can accentuate some of the effects of sex, but don't overdo it.*

HOW TANTRIC ARE YOU NOW?

- ☐ Have you been able to make your partner's body vibrate using your mouth?
- ☐ Have you succeeded in reaching a calm, meditative state using the mantra *So Hum*?
- ☐ Have you succeeded in intoning *OM* both on your own and during sex?
- ☐ Have you used a vibrator on yourself?
- ☐ Have you let your partner watch you using a vibrator on yourself?
- ☐ Have you used a vibrator on your partner?
- ☐ Have you meditated on a ready-made *yantra*?
- ☐ Have you created your own *yantra* from a digital image of your partner's *yoni* or *lingam*?
- ☐ Have you experimented with *pranayama*?
- ☐ Have you co-ordinated slight hyperventilation during sex?

If you answered 'yes' to between eight and ten questions you're obviously very open to Tantric sex ideas and have worked hard on acquiring the skills.

If you answered 'yes' to between five and seven questions you're on your way but you have quite a bit of experimenting and practising to do.

If you couldn't answer 'yes' to more than four questions, read the chapter again and really get down to training your mind and your body. Mantras, *yantras* and breathing exercises are important tools in Tantric sex for reaching *ananda*.

5

Tantric foreplay and massage

In this chapter you will learn:
- *that your partner is a god or goddess*
- *how to perform* nyasa
- *how to sensitize the skin for more powerful orgasms.*

> *Nyasa is necessary for the production of the desired state of mind... Transformation of thought is Transformation of being. This is the essential principle and rational basis of all this and similar Tantrik* sadhana.
>
> Arthur Avalon (Sir John Woodroffe), Introduction to the *Mahanirvana Tantra*

Nyasa is a powerful kind of foreplay that embraces the body, the mind and the spirit by worshipping the woman as literally a goddess and the man as literally a god. Originally, most Tantrikas treated their partners like this only during the ceremony of the *cakrapuja* (see Chapter 3) and after that it was back to normal. Other male Tantrikas considered that a woman was a goddess, or was inhabited by a goddess, all the time. Possibly the most vital part of the Tantric sex I teach is that women *and men* are goddesses and gods *throughout their lives*.

If you think of your partner as a goddess or god, she or he will become a goddess or god.

If there's just one thing you could do to improve not just your sex life but also your entire life together, then it would be adopting this outlook. Many religions teach the idea that God is within, and this is simply the logical application of that belief. But, as I've stressed, you don't need to be at all religious to have spiritual feelings. Let's consider how remarkable every human being is. Here are just three of the ways:

▶ *Every human being is composed of something like 10,000 trillion cells. Even more mind-boggling, every single cell contains literally millions of components, including huge numbers of mitochondria, which are the cell's power sources. Way back in time, mitochondria seem to have been bacteria living quite separately. So you and your partner can be seen not so much as single organisms as vast collections of organisms.*
▶ *Every single atom of which your partner is composed literally came from the stars and has already been in huge numbers of other organisms, because atoms can survive for a million years or more. Do you like to think of your partner as Cleopatra or Mark Antony? Well, quite possibly some part is.*
▶ *At this very moment rays from outer space (cosmic rays – part of the electromagnetic spectrum) are passing right through your partner's body as well as your body. Looking at it in a rather different way, your bodies are always composed, to a tiny extent, of cosmic rays, that therefore connect you to deep space. And when you embrace, the same cosmic rays pass through both of you, so you're both connected to deep space and one another.*

I could continue at length. But you get the idea. Every human being is something quite extraordinary. *Nyasa*, which I'll be explaining in a moment, is the Tantric way of helping us to see our partners as they *truly* are, that is, as incredible manifestations of a *something* that modern science has yet fully to understand. As I've observed before, if you know anything at all about modern techniques for reprogramming the mind, such as cognitive therapy or Neuro-Linguistic Programming (NLP), you'll realize that Tantra was there before. *Nyasa*, you could say, is a way of reprogramming participants to see the divine in every person.

But even if you don't accept any of that, you should still treat your partner with complete respect. Just from an entirely selfish point of view, a confident, happy partner who feels appreciated will be a better lover than someone who has been made to feel anxious and unworthy.

One of the reasons for having random pairings in the left-hand version of the *cakrapuja* (see Chapter 3) was precisely that every man and every woman, irrespective of caste, age or physical appearance, was recognized as a manifestation of the divine. From that point of view, it made no difference with whom you had sex.

Nyasa – the transformative touch

You are about to enter into a world of magic and sensuality in which you take turns to stimulate different parts of one another's bodies. So this isn't like a normal massage in which one person is passive and the other does all the work. You both give and receive pleasure. But *nyasa* goes beyond the physical preparation for *whole body orgasms*. It's also a form of mental reprogramming that helps you relate to your partner in a new and better way, even, perhaps, leading to out of body experiences. Mantra (see previous chapter) can precede *nyasa*, as well as being included in it. At first it all may seem a little weird, but as time goes on and you practise this and other aspects of Tantric sex, so your outlook will gradually change.

▶ **Step 1:** *Prepare by showering, either together or separately, and adorning your naked bodies with whatever accessories you've chosen (see Chapter 11 for more on Tantric accessories).*
▶ **Step 2:** *Sit opposite one another on the bed or somewhere comfortable. One of you gently take hold of your partner's foot. The authentic Tantrikas in the* cakrapuja *would have recited a mantra:* Ang, Kring, Kring, Yang, Rang, Lang, Vang, Shang, Shang, Sang, Hong, Haung, Hangsah; *and then*

followed that by saying something to invite the deity into the body, such as 'The embodied spirit of the highly blessed and auspicious goddess is placed here.' You can do the same if you wish, but you might be more comfortable using OM (see previous chapter) and saying something more natural like, 'This is the beautiful foot of my beautiful goddess/god.' Or, rather than stick to a formula you could simply describe what you see and express appreciation in your own words, such as, 'I love this foot because it's your foot, the foot belonging to my goddess/god...' Or, 'You're my goddess/god and your body drives me wild with desire.' Whatever you say, you should believe it (see Meaning it, p. 94). Now really look at the foot. Notice the shape, the pattern of the veins, which toe is longest... Gently stroke it... Kiss it... Suck the toes in turn, paying special attention to the big toe of the left foot (see p. 96). Separate the toes and very softly caress between them, using a little scented massage oil or cream (see p. 98).

▶ Step 3: *Your partner does the same to you.*

▶ Step 4: *Your partner now selects part of your body and you go through the same kind of ritual, as appropriate. Whatever your partner did to you, you then do the same to your partner.*

▶ Step 5: *At some point you'll find it appropriate to get more intimately close, in which case Shakti can sit on Shiva's lap, facing him with her ankles crossed behind him.*

▶ Step 6: *Continue in the same way, taking the initiative by turns, but leaving the genitals till last. Vary the kind of stimulation. Be imaginative. Don't overlook places like the ears, neck and scalp. You can make massaging movements using the oil or cream but you can also tickle, stroke, pinch, squeeze, slap, pull, scratch, breathe onto, suck, lick, nibble, bite, and so on. While being free to move a little, maintain a harmonious, symmetrical face-to-face pose as far as possible. In other words, don't ask your partner to get on hands and knees so you can admire their buttocks. That destroys the harmony. Rather, slip your hands around or under your partner to caress the buttocks, while remaining face to face.*

▶ Step 7: *When you reach the genitals, first of all spend plenty of time admiring them. Constantly changing in colour, size and shape according to the degree of engorgement, they're an endless source of fascination, especially when you reflect that your partner's genitals were made from the same basic kinds of tissues as your own (see Table 5.1). When you've finished looking you can stimulate them with your fingers or perform* auparishtaka *as described in the next chapter.*

The early Tantrikas would have followed a very specific ritual. This more flexible approach allows you to make *nyasa* different each time, and to be creative. It's a great opportunity not only to discover your partner's most erogenous zones but also the most effective way to stimulate them. And by taking turns it also becomes slightly easier for either of you to 'ask' for what you want. For example, if you would like your partner to suck one of your nipples you only have to suck your partner's nipple first.

Meaning it

As we saw in Chapter 2, where the mind goes the energy follows. Up until this moment, for example, you probably weren't consciously aware of your underwear against your genitals. Now you are. 'Meaning it' is a related concept. In other words, it's no good doing these things in an offhand, mechanical sort of way. There won't be any effect. If you take hold of your partner's hand in a perfunctory manner, you'll only communicate disinterest. But do exactly the same with the intention to communicate affection and your partner will sense it.

This is part of what I meant by my use of the word 'magic' earlier on. You have to put your mind into whatever you're doing or saying. If you regularly practice *nyasa* (and you can do it in a small way every day) so you'll come to see your partner differently.

It's unfortunate that once the original walking-on-air feeling has gone out of a relationship, it's so often replaced by a struggle for superiority. Even worse, it's not even a positive competition for self-improvement but a negative, destructive battle in which the most dominant boosts his or her ego by putting the other person down whenever possible.

When you think about it, it's completely crazy. Two people see wonderful things in one another and then set about destroying the very qualities they found attractive. *Nyasa* is one way of reversing that. Don't knock your partner down, build him or her up. When you say that your partner is a goddess or god, say it with feeling. And day by day you'll come to realize that it's true.

Massage techniques

Effleurage is a French word denoting a soothing, stroking action which works well on the back. Sitting on your partner's lap, or with your partner sitting on your lap, reach under your partner's arms and, with your hands covered in warm massage oil or cream, put one hand each side of your partner's spine and glide steadily up. When you've gone as far as you can reach, then, with very light pressure only, glide your hands out and back down along your partner's sides to the starting position. Repeat several times.

Kneading is a technique to use on tense muscles. The shoulders are a great place to start. At the end of *effleurage*, move both hands to one shoulder, pick up the muscle in one hand, squeeze it gently, then push it towards the other hand. The new hand then also kneads the muscle before pushing it back. In this way, the muscle is worked rhythmically between the two hands. Once you've done one shoulder, turn your attention to the other.

Two fingers (the pads of your index and middle fingers) can be used to make small circular movements. Work your way up from the base of the spine to the neck, doing both sides simultaneously. You can also work on the muscles.

The big toe

Some yogis and Tantrikas consider the big toe of the left foot to be highly erotic. Intriguingly, modern science has revealed that the areas of the brain concerned with the genitals and with the toes are next to one another. It seems possible that activity in one area can overflow into the other. There may also be an explanation in the fact that the nerve serving the foot and the nerve serving the penis and clitoris merge at the sacral plexus.

This idea was picked up by Emanuel Swedenborg (1688–1772), the Swedish mystic and scientist, who wrote in his *Spiritual Diary* about the way 'fire' in his penis also caused a stream of fire 'into the big toe of the left foot, and...especially into the nail of the big toe of the left foot, which at length co-responds with a fiery burning of such a kind in the glans penis...'

Swedenborg's writings in turn inspired the poet and artist William Blake (1757–1827), an early English seeker after Tantric knowledge, to produce a daring engraving of himself with a flaming star descending to his left foot and with his penis erect.

Indisputably, there are huge numbers of nerve endings in the feet and learning how to massage them can give your partner enormous pleasure. Taking the big toe of your partner's left foot into your mouth and sucking it from top to bottom is a winning way to start.

Insight
In the late 1940s in America, Kinsey found that couples with 'low educational attainment' spent very little time on foreplay

while those with a higher education spent 12 minutes. By
the mid-1970s Morton Hunt found that foreplay was about
15 minutes, irrespective of education. I'd suggest foreplay
should last at least double that for a proper Tantric session, with
the part devoted to *nyasa* lasting 15 minutes as a minimum.

The supreme deity

Many Tantrikas see the supreme deity as being both male
and female and there are innumerable statues depicting
this very thing, a double-sexed being with an erect penis
and a woman's breast, known as *Ardhanari*. As it says in
the *Navaratnesvara*: 'She who is absolute Being, Bliss and
Consciousness may be thought of as female, male or neuter
Brahman although, in reality, she is none of these.'

According to this view, the supreme deity split into male
and female parts. In the same way, we humans, too, are
only 'halves', which is why we feel lonely, and will never be
complete until we unite entirely with our partners. Many
people do feel that.

Tantrikas also believe that every man contains a female
aspect and every woman a male aspect, with the left side
of the body being female and the right male.

Men's and women's bodies are actually far more similar than most
people realize. In fact, male and female embryos are anatomically
identical during the first weeks of development. At six to seven
weeks the foetus looks essentially female with no external genitals
other than a tiny protuberance called the 'genital tubercle'. It's only
from this point on that the difference becomes obvious, with the
genital tubercle developing either as the clitoris or as the head, or

glans, of the penis. In fact, male and female sex organs are derived from the same kinds of tissues, as the table below shows:

Table 5.1 Sex organs from the same kinds of embryonic tissue

Men	Women
Testes	Ovaries
Penis	Clitoral system
Penile glans	Clitoral glans
Foreskin	Clitoral hood
Scrotum	Labia majora
Cowper's glands	Bartholin's glands

So by playing around with your own body you can, to a meaningful extent, get an idea of how things will feel to your partner.

Oils and creams for *nyasa*

Oils or creams make an amazing difference to *nyasa,* both for the giver and the receiver. The whole experience becomes far more pleasurable and sensual for both.

But which should you choose? Oil is usually the cheapest and also the most natural option, especially if you select something from the kitchen. Any light vegetable oil such as sunflower, safflower or grapeseed is fine. Almond oil is especially good and comes with a pleasant, natural scent.

You can also create scents with a few drops of essential oils, available from health shops. Rose, musk, ylang ylang, orchid, vanilla and cinnamon are all sexy. You don't have to stick with just one. Try creating your own special scent by combining them. Never apply essential oils directly to the skin – they're highly concentrated and could, at that strength, even be harmful.

Buy your massage oils in small quantities and store them in a cool place, in the dark, tightly closed – once they oxidize they smell rancid and will no longer create pleasure. Pour the quantity you're going to be using into an attractive bowl, add the chosen essential oil or oils, and warm it (by, for example, standing the bowl in a basin of hot water). Using cold oil on the skin creates exactly the opposite of the effect that you want.

The disadvantage of oil is that it tends to be messy (especially if you knock the bowl over) and isn't easily absorbed into the skin. Creams, on the other hand, are specially formulated for quick absorption, are much easier to handle in a bedroom situation and won't cause a mess if knocked over. Their disadvantage is that they can be expensive, can be packed full of all kinds of 'artificial' chemicals and aren't easy to warm up, other than by rubbing a quantity between the hands.

I'd recommend a massage cream for *nyasa*, oil for body to body techniques (see below).

> **Tip:** It's generally best to keep massage oils and creams away from the genitals and to use artificial lubricants in those areas (see p. 100). In particular, oil can make holes in latex condoms.

Advanced *nyasa*

When parts of your partner's body are not very responsive, regular *nyasa* will gradually increase the number of nerve endings. You can accelerate this 'training' by linking the unresponsive part with your partner's genitals and by making erotic suggestions.

- ▶ **Step 1:** *Begin* nyasa *as usual until you come to the body part that's unresponsive.*
- ▶ **Step 2:** *Stimulate your partner's genitals using an artificial lubricant (see below).*

▶ **Step 3:** *Stimulate the unresponsive body part three times in whatever way is most appropriate (licking, pinching, circling or whatever).*

▶ **Step 4:** *Stimulate your partner's genitals three times.*

▶ **Step 5:** *Alternate Steps 3 and 4 for a few minutes, keeping up the three-time rhythm so your partner knows three stimulations of the unresponsive part will always be followed by three highly-pleasurable stimulations of the genitals. At the same time you can add in verbal suggestions such as, 'Whenever I touch you here you'll know I'm going to masturbate you afterwards.'*

The psychological conditioning of the body can happen quite quickly but physical changes can take months to be noticed. Of course, you can also use the same technique on yourself if you're dissatisfied with the lack of response from a part of your own body.

Lubricants for ecstasy

If you were to ask me one quick, easy thing you could do to increase the ecstatic power of sex I'd say buy an artificial lubricant. Like oils and creams, artificial lubricants can also be used all over the body, but it's applied to the *lingam* and *yoni* that they work their most powerful magic. Both men and women produce natural lubricants, of course, and they're normally sufficient to allow comfortable sex. But the right artificial lubricants do much more than that. They can:

▶ *increase sensuality and sensitivity*

▶ *change the quality of the stimulation*

▶ *let sex continue longer*

▶ *protect the* yonis *of older women*

▶ *make less responsive areas more responsive (for example, the perineum and scrotum)*

▶ *lubricate areas that don't produce anything naturally (for example, for sliding the* lingam *back and forth between the breasts or thighs).*

There are three main types:

▶ *Oil-based lubricants. These have tended to fall out of favour, partly because they can damage latex condoms.*
▶ *Silicone lubricants. The advantage is that they don't evaporate and remain extremely slippery for extended periods. Some people report that the silicone dulls sexual response – which can be an advantage in some circumstances, a disadvantage in others.*
▶ *Water-based lubricants. Some brands have the consistency of natural lubrication while others are thicker and yet others, such as KY jelly, are gels. Apart from their natural feel, the advantage of water-based lubricants is that traces on sheets are easily washed away. The disadvantage is that water-based lubricants do dry out after a while. Of course, you can easily add more but a fun (and cheaper) solution is to 'refresh' the lubricant with a little water. Put some warm water into an indoor plant sprayer before sex and keep it close. When you feel the need, spray your own genitals and your partner's – apart from anything else it feels very nice.*

Although you'll find a restricted range of lubricants in most chemists, a sex shop will give you the best choice. If you're frightened about going in, go in anyway – you would then be breaking a taboo in the authentic Tantric fashion (see Chapter 3). Online sex shops will also have a big range (but that's not so daring). If you've never used artificial lubricants before, I'd suggest buying small amounts of three different types to compare. You may well find that one type of lubricant actually spoils sex as far as you're concerned and it would be a pity to be put off lubricants entirely by that.

Insight

A great 'trick' is to put some silicone or water-based lubricant into the teat of the condom before putting it on. When the *lingam* is moving inside the *yoni* the lubricant will gradually flood out of the teat, creating a sensation not unlike the flood of a woman's natural lubrication. Don't forget that oil-based

(Contd)

lubricant shouldn't be used with latex condoms as it can cause the latex to break down. However, if you're using the slightly thinner and more sensitive polyurethane condoms you can use oil-based lubricants if you wish.

If you're going to be enjoying *auparishtaka* (oral sex) which is the subject of the next chapter, you probably won't want to apply any lubricant right now.

SHAVING

Tantric art shows genitals that are completely shaven, *yonis* that are shaven only around the labia, and genitals that are not shaven at all. As for the texts, some refer to *yonis* ringed with hair but it's not clear if that means in their natural state or with the hair shaven or plucked around the opening so as literally to leave a 'frame'. So it's really up to you.

As part of *nyasa* you might occasionally attend to one another's pubic locks. The easiest and safest way is to use a specially designed 'woman's' electric razor. Don't use a man's beard trimmer because it can trap and cut loose skin. It's best to do this before showering – you can then hose away the cut hairs that otherwise would be annoying in *auparishtaka* (oral sex – see next chapter).

Insight

Shaktis, if you want to excite your Shiva, you'll almost certainly find that a clear view of a shaven *yoni* will have a powerful effect. Shivas, you're unlikely to find your Shakti is any more or less excited by the extent of your pubic hair but trimming it will make your *lingam* appear longer. It will also make fellatio more agreeable for your partner. Both of you should find that shaving makes the skin more sensitive (men should include their scrotums).

Oxytocin – the orgasmic chemical

Some lovers, men particularly, may think *nyasa* is rather boring and be anxious to get onto the 'main action'. On the contrary, performing *nyasa* is a vital step in creating the altered state of mind that is the aim of Tantric sex – and it can lead to more powerful orgasms, too.

The fact is that strange things happen when you have skin contact with your lover. The cause is oxytocin. Oxytocin is a peptide secreted by the pituitary gland, which promotes affection, bonding, touching and cuddling, sensitizes the skin and, indeed, makes sex more enjoyable.

Oxytocin is an extraordinary drug. It does wonderful things and, since you make it yourself, it's completely legal. No one can stop you. Yet it's more powerful than many illegal substances. Here's what it can do for you:

▶ *makes the skin sensitive to touch*
▶ *increases the sensitivity of the* lingam *and clitoris*
▶ *probably encourages women to display their* yonis *and to desire penetration*
▶ *is responsible for orgasmic contractions*
▶ *promotes feelings of affection*
▶ *increases various other chemicals such as dopamine and serotonin which increase happiness*
▶ *impairs reasoning and memory so that nothing seems to matter.*

Insight

The impairment of reasoning and memory seems, at first sight, to be a rather weird and inexplicable side-effect of oxytocin. One theory is that, being released in large quantities during childbirth, it helps women forget the pain (and, therefore, be willing to go through the whole

(Contd)

thing again and again). My theory is that in sex one of its functions is to put things into perspective. Have you ever noticed, for example, how after a good sex session you can barely remember the things about your partner that had been annoying you? And if you can just remember, how those things no longer seem at all important? Which they probably weren't. That's oxytocin.

Have a go

Fifteen minutes of *nyasa* will considerably increase oxytocin. This 'supertouching' causes the person doing it to experience a huge surge.

▶ **Step 1:** *You can do this while sitting face to face as part of* nyasa *or, for the maximum effect, have your partner lie on the bed or floor and, straddling their thighs, kneel comfortably and sit down on their legs. Both of you should, of course, be naked for which the room should be at a comfortable temperature.*

▶ **Step 2:** *If you've already performed* nyasa *for five or ten minutes go straight to the next step. Otherwise, rub your hands together to warm them up, take a little of your selected massage oil or cream (see p. 98) and rub it between your hands to warm it, and then give your partner a short massage, to awaken their skin and your hands.*

▶ **Step 3:** *This is the key part. Place the tips of the three middle fingers of each hand very lightly on your partner's sides just below the armpits and with your eyes closed draw them very, very slowly along the contours of your partner's body down to the thighs. Particularly focus on your forefingers. There should be virtually no friction so that your fingertips glide at a steady pace. If they judder use more massage oil or cream. The speed should be such that, if you open your eyes for a moment, you can barely detect the movement. Imagine that your partner's skin cells are, like paving stones, separated by cracks and that you're aiming to detect every one of them.*

▶ **Step 4:** *Say to yourself that you're touching the skin of a goddess/god.*

▶ **Step 5:** *Switch roles so you can both benefit equally from the oxytocin hit.*

BODY TO BODY NYASA

In this form of *nyasa*, rather than use only your hands, you're going to use your entire bodies to stimulate one another. This, therefore, resembles the more erotic versions of the Japanese *nuru* ('slippery') massage, which uses a gel made from seaweed. But massage oil or body lotion will do almost as well (cream isn't slippery enough).

▶ **Step 1:** *This is going to be extremely messy so you're going to need to protect your bedding – as the very minimum, put a couple of old sheets over it.*

▶ **Step 2:** *While your partner is lying face downwards, massage a generous quantity of oil all over the legs, back and buttocks, keeping in mind that she/he is a goddess/god. Spread oil on your chest and lay down on top. Rub your chest all over your partner's back, remembering that you, too, are a goddess/god.*

▶ **Step 3:** *Spread a generous quantity of oil on your own buttocks and sit on your partner's buttocks. Move your buttocks round and round, from side to side, backwards and forwards and in a figure-of-eight. Slide backwards and forwards along your partner's back. Slide your perineum up and down your partner's legs (if you're a woman you may be able to orgasm this way, if you wish).*

▶ **Step 4:** *With both of you smothered in oil, just writhe about on one another in every way you can think of. By all means use your hands, too, but concentrate on the idea of this being a body-to-body massage. Be inventive and uninhibited. Try to feel every part of your own body and every part of your partner's body.*

MASSAGE FOR SEXUAL HEALTH

Everybody knows about the circulation of the blood. Less well known is the circulation of lymphatic fluid that fights disease, eliminates toxins and shifts fat. The lymphatic system has no pump; it relies entirely on activity of the muscles. In other words, if you're not getting much exercise, your lymphatic system may get clogged up.

This is where a therapeutic massage can help. Warm up with a basic massage, giving plenty of *effleurage*. Then introduce the additional technique of intermittent pressure. Lymph fluid is what's known as 'thixotropic'. That's to say that it can exist in either a liquid or a gel form. When you press hard it turns to gel and doesn't move easily. So, you have to push gently with your fingers and palms, both downwards and in the direction the lymph needs to travel from the hands towards the shoulders and from the feet towards the groin. Push several times before moving on.

There are several lymph nodes situated in the crease between the thigh and the abdomen. In a healthy person, one or more can just be felt, like little peas below the surface. If they're enlarged or painful then a blockage is indicated. Gently work your way along from the genitals up the crease towards the hip bone. (This is something you can do for yourself if your partner isn't available.) Then, from the middle of the crease work your way diagonally up towards the navel and then straight up to the breast bone.

If you're not going to have sex, there's an excellent way of ending the massage that involves building tension throughout the body then abruptly releasing it. At an agreed moment, the person doing the massaging ceases all touching, and their partner takes several deep breaths then holds one breath and clenches every possible muscle for ten seconds. It helps to raise the legs, arms and torso for maximum tension. The partner then completely relaxes and breathes normally. The effect is enhanced if he or she wears an eye mask and if there's some soft music playing.

10 THINGS TO REMEMBER

1   Nyasa *is a powerful kind of foreplay that embraces body, mind and spirit.*

2   *If you treat your partner as a goddess/god he or she will become a goddess/god.*

3   Nyasa *is an ancient technique for influencing the mind, just as powerful as modern techniques such as cognitive therapy and Neuro-Linguistic Programming (NLP).*

4   *You have to put your mind into the things you're doing and saying and really mean them if the 'magic' is to be effective.*

5   *Men's and women's bodies are far more similar than most people realize, which means you can, to a considerable extent, test things on yourself before trying them with your partner.*

6   *Massage cream will make* nyasa *far more sensual.*

7   *It's possible to 'train' less responsive parts of the body to become more sensitive over time.*

8   *Artificial lubricants are to be preferred for the genital region but they can also be used all over the body.*

9   *Displaying a shaven* yoni *is hugely exciting to most men; men should also at least trim their pubic hair.*

10   *Oxytocin, a chemical released by skin to skin contact, sensitizes the genitals and makes orgasms more powerful.*

HOW TANTRIC ARE YOU NOW?

☐ Have you and your partner performed *nyasa* together?
☐ Have you discovered any erogenous zones on your partner's body that you didn't know about, or found a new way of stimulating an area that you did know about?
☐ Are you thinking of your partner as a goddess/god and behaving accordingly?
☐ Are you spending at least half an hour on *nyasa* and other kinds of foreplay?
☐ Have you succeeded in 'training' any part of your partner's body, or your own body, to be more sensitive?
☐ Have you shaven or at least trimmed one another's pubic hair?
☐ Have you tried 'supertouching' on p. 104?
☐ Have you tried body to body massage and gone really wild?
☐ Have you noticed the oxytocin buzz?
☐ Have you given your partner a massage for sexual health?

If you answered 'yes' to between eight and ten questions you're obviously very open to Tantric sex ideas and have worked hard on acquiring the skills.

If you answered 'yes' to between five and seven questions you're on your way but you have quite a bit of experimenting and practising to do.

If you couldn't answer 'yes' to more than four questions, maybe you're thinking that *nyasa* sounds rather dull or silly. In that case, read the chapter again and at least give it all a go. You may be very surprised by the results.

6

Auparishtaka – Tantric oral sex

In this chapter you will learn:
- *why the early Tantrikas believed sex was magic*
- *how to please your goddess with cunnilingus*
- *how to please your god with fellatio.*

> *The man who is going to have sex with a woman should*
> *drink the nectar of her tongue in the mouth...*
>
> The *Kaulavalinirnaya*

Oral sex was incredibly important to the early Tantrikas. But
they had a rather unusual way of going about it, as we'll see
in a moment. For them it meant gnosis (that is, the intuitive
understanding of spiritual truths), magical powers and a sense
of oneness. No educated person today would subscribe to the first
two, but the third remains important. I'll be explaining how you
can adapt the Tantric rituals to create your own very special and
intimate oneness with your partner.

The extraordinary true history of Tantric sex

Let's say you had been living in India as a Tantrika around fifteen
hundred years ago. Let's say you believed in magic, which you
would have done in that era. And let's suppose that, for whatever

reason, you wanted something that could give you magical powers. What might you have done? Sought out a guru who could impart a secret spell? Maybe. Gone to a herbalist to buy a plant that caused an altered mental state? Maybe. What about acquiring a liquid that was actually *proven* to have the power of life? Wouldn't that trump everything?

The early Tantrikas didn't know about sperm and they didn't know about ova – how could they? – but they did know there was something incredible about the fluids produced by men and women (*especially* women) during sex. They knew they had the power to create life, to create human form, out of something that resembled water. So, in my words, their thinking went something like this:

> *All life flows ultimately from the womb of the Goddess. Women bring forth life which, therefore, also indirectly comes from the womb of the Goddess. Unlike a man, a woman's sexual fluids flow, to a greater or lesser extent, all the time. A woman is therefore continuously flowing with the power of the Goddess.*

As we saw earlier, it was believed that there were semi-divine *yoginis* who, existing as pure spirit, could inhabit the bodies of real women so as to have sex with men during the *Kaula* ceremony of the *cakrapuja*. Therefore, women's sexual fluids were especially magical if consumed when they were taken over by the *yoginis*, that is, during sex. What's more, since it was known that it was the combination of the woman's and the man's sexual fluids that produced life, so drinking the combined fluids was even more potent. Originally, then, Tantric sex was simply *the means of producing magical, sexual fluids*.

Nowadays, even with the wonders of the electron microscope to reveal full details of the miracle of life, we're far more blasé about semen and ova than we should be. We know so many of the secrets we're no longer awed. But people were once.

Tantra and magic

According to Abhinavagupta in the *Tantraloka*, the mouth (by which he meant the *yoni*) is the most important chakra. 'How could consciousness itself,' he asked, 'be conveyed by writing?' In other words, the reality of the universe is something that can only be apprehended intuitively and the consumption of a woman's sexual fluids was one of the ways. But the Tantrikas also had worldly goals in addition to the spiritual.

The eighth century *Hevajra Tantra*, which is Buddhist, says a man should drink his semen mixed with *adharamadhu* ('the honey down below') in order to gain *siddhis* (magical powers) including the ability to fly and even immortality. Tantras ever since have promised much the same.

None wanted magical powers more than the aristocracy. Many already considered themselves to be semi-divine and the idea of having sex, even by proxy, with goddesses and gods, and of acquiring their powers, was intoxicating. (At the same time, the idea that 'ordinary' people might acquire magical powers must have been somewhat threatening.)

The *siddhis* included:

- ▶ *power over the elements*
- ▶ *the ability to grow larger or smaller*
- ▶ *invisibility*
- ▶ *the ability to enter into another person's body*
- ▶ *the power to make others subservient*
- ▶ *the power to torment or kill an opponent at a distance*
- ▶ *erasing bad* **karma** *from a previous incarnation*
- ▶ *longevity or immortality*
- ▶ *flight (see factbox, p. 112).*

Although the emphasis gradually shifted to sex itself, there are still those for whom the fluid remains the source of magic, in Puri,

Orissa, for example, and among the Nizarpanthis of Western India, who make a dish called *payal* with semen.

Flight

The power of flight was one of the *siddhis* that was most sought after. According to various sources, including the eighth century *Malati-Madhava*, it could be powered by the five 'nectars' which, in this case, were said to be semen, blood, urine, excrement and bone marrow. In the *Kathasaritsagara* of Somadeva, Queen Kuvalayavali, describes how she 'suddenly saw that my friends, having taken off, were gliding about in the sky'. Calling to them to come down, she demanded to know the secret and was told that 'the supernatural power' came from 'eating human flesh' – a rather extreme way of consuming the nectars.

But did people really believe that flying was possible? Surely they must have noticed that nobody ever actually succeeded? These are difficult questions to answer. But we only have to look at some of the beliefs held in our own time to know that otherwise sane people can convince themselves of the most extraordinary things.

There is, however, another explanation and that is the Tantric belief in the subtle body (discussed in Chapter 2). Yes, the physical body remained on the ground. But that didn't matter because the subtle body, which was just as real, temporarily left the physical body and flew where it pleased. The *Rig Veda* says that, 'Among all the things that fly, the mind is the swiftest.' And the *Kalingabodhi Jataka* says that flying involves 'clothing the body with the raiment of contemplation.' No doubt alcohol and hallucinatory drugs played a part. But it also seems to be the case that while we dismiss dreams as, at most, indications of our unconscious thoughts, the early Tantrikas found them as equally valid as their other mental states.

Menstrual blood

The early Tantrikas also had an ingenious line of reasoning about menstrual blood which went something like this:

When a woman is nursing a baby she produces milk, but when she is not she produces menstrual blood. Menstrual blood must therefore be a transformation of the breast milk that nourishes a baby and is therefore an especially powerful kind of sexual fluid. Therefore, I will consume menstrual blood.

The *Manthanabhairava Tantra* recommends as a 'secret without equal' that breast milk and menstrual blood (*dharamrtam*) should be mixed together. And the *Kaulajnananirnaya* of Matsyendranatha instructs that 'one should constantly drink blood and semen' directly out of the vulva. Essentially, menstrual blood was a living stream connecting the woman, and through her the *kula* or clan, with the stars.

But menstruation also had its frightening aspects. Because women lost blood it was assumed they also needed to consume blood. It was this that made the goddesses so terrifying and was why a man needed to be a *vira* (hero) to risk intercourse with them.

Warning: Syphilis, gonorrhoea, AIDS, chlamydia and other illnesses can be transmitted by the various oral sex practises described in this chapter. Oral sex is not safe sex. If you have any doubts about the sexual health of your partner, do not engage in either oral sex or intercourse. Suggest to your partner that you should both have check-ups and then follow whatever advice you are given.

Tantric oral sex today – your own *kula*

Since we know perfectly well that people can't fly or acquire any of the other *siddhis*, you may well feel that bodily fluids are something you'd rather leave out of your Tantric sex repertoire. What would be the point? There's a clue in one of the names given to the sexual fluids. Sometimes they were simply *dravyam* (fluid) or *yonitattva* (vulval essence) but also very significantly *kuladravyam* (clan fluid). As we saw in Chapter 3, one of the aims of the *cakrapuja* was to create a '*kula* (clan) feeling' and the drinking of the sexual fluids from the 'alpha couple' was part of that. By consuming something from one another's bodies you'd be helping create your own '*kula*' of two people.

Forget the magic. That's of historical interest only. What you're left with is something worthwhile. It's that sense of uniting your physical bodies as far as you possibly can. Of being as intimate as you can. Of reconnecting male and female. Of abolishing loneliness. Of becoming one.

Have a go
Perhaps you sometimes say things like 'I could eat you' as an expression of endearment and love. Well, now you can prove it. How far you want to go is up to you.

▶ **Step 1:** *Prepare a single glass of wine (or whatever you prefer) by adding to it something from your own bodies. If you find the idea of drinking something from your partner actually rather exciting you might like to follow one of the Tantric 'recipes', or you could be more symbolic by, for example, adding flakes of dry skin. My suggestion would be that you each lick a forefinger rather provocatively and use it to stir the wine.*
▶ **Step 2:** *Share the drink, taking alternate sips, while reflecting on the fact that some part of your partner's body is now inside you.*

Some people are quite squeamish about bodily fluids. If that includes you, just keep in mind that there's a huge difference between waste products and other kinds of bodily secretions.

Tantric kissing

Whether or not you like the idea of deliberately consuming bodily fluids, we all *do* consume them as a side-product of our sexual activities. Let's start with the commonest way – kissing. Women tend to like it quite a lot whereas men rather cut it short to move on to other things. That's a mistake because, well done, it can be extremely exciting.

The sixteenth century *Kaulavalinirnaya* of Jnanananda Paramahamsa says that a man who is going to have sex should first drink the 'nectar' of the woman's 'tongue in the mouth'. The ambiguity of Tantric texts leaves open the possibility that the 'tongue' is, in fact, the clitoris but it's probably correct to interpret this on both levels.

Have a go
▶ **Step 1:** *While you're kissing make a point of sucking in and swallowing your partner's saliva. If you're put off by that idea, reflect that we all produce about one to one-and-a-half litres of saliva a day which we swallow and reabsorb. So a little of your partner's saliva is trivial from that point of view. In any event, saliva is 99.5 per cent water and perfectly safe as long as your partner is healthy – in fact, it even contains an anti-bacterial enzyme called lysozyme.*
▶ **Step 2:** *Get busy with those tongues. Rub your tongues against one another and push them into one another's mouths.*
▶ **Step 3:** *Get your partner to push out his or her tongue as far as possible, take it into your mouth and gently suck and bite it. Then swap roles.*
▶ **Step 4:** *Take a mouthful of wine (or any other drink) swallow a little and kiss the rest into your partner's mouth.*
▶ **Step 5:** *Pass food from mouth to mouth. I'm not suggesting you go as far as the* cakrapuja, *when food was prepared with semen and vaginal fluid. But sharing food in an intimate way can be very arousing. The minimum is to take half of something long into your mouth (bread stick, biscuit, asparagus spear etc.) and let your partner eat the other half until your lips meet. But that's still not very Tantric. More authentic would be to*

take some food into your mouth, chew it, bite a piece off and swallow it, then kiss the remainder into your partner's mouth, continuing like this back and forth until all of it is gone.

The tongue

The tongue is, in fact, far more erotic than most people realize because it's served by an incredible five pairs of cranial nerves:

▶ *trigeminal – pain, heat, cold, touch*
▶ *facial – taste at the front of the tongue*
▶ *glossopharyngeal – taste at the rear of the tongue*
▶ *vagus – swallowing movements of the tongue*
▶ *hypoglossal – all muscular movements of the tongue.*

It's not surprising, therefore, that sucking and biting your partner's tongue during intercourse adds considerably to arousal. Nevertheless, with the correct mental focus, it can also be used as a way of taking attention away from the genitals and thus delaying orgasm/ejaculation (for more on this, see Chapter 7).

Cunnilingus

More than anything, the earliest Tantric sex rituals were all about female sexual fluids. But no rational person today believes them to have magical properties in the way it was once thought. So where does that leave us in terms of modern Tantric sex practice?

In fact, given that the aim is to reach the ultimate degree of rapture, cunnilingus cannot be missed out. It:

▶ *increases intimacy*
▶ *prepares the yoni for intercourse*

- *allows a man to give unlimited pleasure*
- *excites the man with the scent and taste of the yoni*
- *allows a man to 'serve' his 'goddess'.*

There's little description of cunnilingus techniques in the *Tantras* but we do have a medieval Tamil poem called the *Kamapanacastiram* (Treatise on the Arrow of Lust) which will do very well. It tells the man to spread his tongue, lick the *yoni* and lap the juices like a 'thirsty dog'. Next, he should make ever-smaller circling movements with his tongue until, opening the inner labia, he should plunge it inside 'like a spear'. He should then continue to explore with his tongue while pressing his nose against the **yonimani** (clitoris). Next, he should take the *yonimani* between his teeth and his tongue and suck it like 'an infant at the breast' until it swells 'like a large ruby'. Finally, he should drink the mixture of his own semen and her fluid which is described as 'rejuvenating'.

Most people will probably want to leave out the last part (drinking the combined sexual fluids from the vagina is known as 'felching' in modern parlance) but the rest is still pretty good advice. Nevertheless, there are a few improvements that could be suggested.

Have a go
- **Step 1:** *Assuming that you're in bed, put a pillow under your goddess's buttocks so that, lying between her open thighs, you have easy access to her yoni. (Sometimes you might like to employ the 69 position for mutual pleasuring but that can be distracting for both of you – you'll undoubtedly create more excitement for your partner if you focus exclusively on her.)*
- **Step 2:** *You might begin by tantalizing her vulva with some heavy breathing (but don't actually blow air into the vagina – it's dangerous).*
- **Step 3:** *Work up from some gentle licks here and there to a firmer full-length tonguing from end to end.*
- **Step 4:** *Take her inner labia into your mouth one at a time and gently play with them.*

▶ **Step 5:** *Move to the clitoris, the primary source of a woman's sexual pleasure. It actually contains some 8,000 nerve fibres, double the number in a penis, so it can cause some pretty explosive effects if you know what to do with it. Nowadays, most women and men can locate it but there are still quite a few who don't realize that it has a hood, analogous to the male foreskin, which hides the really exciting part, known as the glans. It's the hood and the shaft that normally get stimulated during cunnilingus and that's where you should begin with gentle, slow licks building to maximum speed.*

▶ **Step 6:** *If you really want to give your partner a cosmic experience you need to expose that glans and get to work on it. You can do that by putting one hand on the mons and gently moving the skin up towards the navel. That will have the effect of retracting the hood of the clitoris and you'll then see a tiny almost translucent red organ which, in most women, is about the size of a lentil. That glans is extremely sensitive. Some women may even find it so delicate they can't stand any direct contact with it. But, most women, having already been aroused, will find a tongue on their exposed glans an ecstatic experience.*

▶ **Step 7:** *Move to the entrance to the vagina. Penetrate again and again with your tongue as far as you possibly can. Explore with circling movements.*

▶ **Step 8:** *Your Shakti may enjoy having her anus included. In fact, she certainly will if she's sufficiently uninhibited because it's absolutely packed with nerve endings. (For more on this see Chapter 9.)*

These are just guidelines. Every woman is different, so it's important to be sensitive to your partner's reactions and pay attention to those little noises of contentment or discomfort. If in doubt, ask (but if you have a lot of questions save them for later rather than break the mood). And, of course, don't go through the same routine mechanically every time. Your aim should be to give your partner at least one orgasm this way.

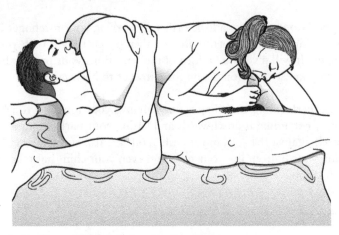

Figure 6.1 *Cunnilingus and fellatio in the 69 position* (Auparishtaka).

Tongue training

As we saw in Chapter 3, some Tantrikas deliberately severed the lingual frenum so they could perform *khechari mudra*. I would certainly not recommend doing anything to damage the tongue in any way but, like many parts of the body, its performance can certainly be improved through training. In fact, there are yogis who can extend their tongues as far as their eyebrows. That would certainly make them unusual lovers, but if you can push your tongue inside the entrance of your partner's *yoni* that's quite enough to give her the exciting sensation of being penetrated.

Extend your tongue in front of a mirror. How far can you stick it out? It usually feels a lot further than it actually is. So set yourself a target and practise regularly.

For effective *yoni* penetration you need to be able to stick your tongue out in a straight line, not curving downwards. Again, watch in the mirror and practise.

A good tip is to make a little orifice by curving your forefinger against the side of your thumb, and then penetrating it with your tongue. It will give you an idea of the sensations your partner feels when you use your tongue on the entrance to her vagina.

When performing cunnilingus you can give your tongue a rest by simply extending it downwards and letting your partner grind herself against the soft, moist flesh. You can also stimulate her by using your bottom lip, your nose and even your chin (but take care with stubble).

Pheromones

Among scientists there's some controversy over whether or not women produce pheromones (chemical signals) and, if they do, whether or not men can detect them. Personally, I'm convinced. But whether it's pheromones, or whether it's simply natural scent, the fact is that when a woman is excited, a man is automatically aroused by her perfume. So that's another very important reason for performing cunnilingus.

Insight

I'll never forget the first time I saw a young stallion catch the scent of a mare on heat. The effect was electric and, quite frankly, terrifying. That day I saw the undeniable power of pheromones at work as the animal rose up on its hind legs, casting its handler aside like a twig, snorting like a steam engine, its penis as instantly hard as an iron bar. Pheromones are a language that you should learn to 'speak' and understand.

EATING FROM THE YONI

Some men quite like the idea not only of taking food from their partner's mouths but also from the 'lower mouth' or *yoni*.

It's very intimate and another way of following the Tantric practice of consuming sexual fluids. The rules are that nothing should be inserted that might:

▶ *get 'lost' inside*
▶ *break and leave a crumb inside*
▶ *irritate or sting*
▶ *create a susceptibility to thrush (i.e. nothing sweet or sugary).*

Possibilities include peeled carrots, well-washed celery and smooth bread sticks. Assuming your partner is agreeable, just 'dip' them into the entrance of her *yoni* and consume as an appetizer.

TIPS FOR SHAKTIS

In my focus groups women sometimes complain that their partners aren't very good at cunnilingus. The way to make a man better is to guide him, firstly, by using 'informal mantras' (see Chapter 4). That's to say, moan and groan ecstatically when it feels nice. That's always very encouraging. Also, writhe around a little (but not so much that he can't keep on target). And, in addition to the 'informal mantras' say exactly what you want. Don't be embarrassed. But there's a very important rule: *Never say anything critical.*

Always find a positive way to express things. So don't say, 'You've missed my clitoris again.' Instead, say, 'You drive me wild when you lick a little bit higher.' Nowadays, most men like to 'give' their partners as many orgasms as possible. It makes men feel proud. So don't be backwards. Explain the secrets of your body (which, after all, a man can't know otherwise). And if you'd like more (or less), say that too. Your partner's reward will come from you *showing* your excitement in every way.

In the previous chapter I suggested shaving one another as part of *nyasa*. Most men seem to prefer a clear view of the *yoni* and, from the woman's point of view, it increases the sensitivity of the skin.

According to one yarn, the fifth Dalai Lama, who died around 1680, was being criticized by his advisers because of his womanizing. In answer he urinated from one of the upper terraces of the palace. The stream of urine ran down the walls to the ground...then re-ascended and re-entered his penis and bladder.

On the face of it, it's no more than a story to demonstrate that the Dalai Lama was an extraordinary being who could not be judged by society's ordinary standards. But there's more to it than that. The Dalai Lama was showing off his prowess at *vajroli mudra* that is, the ability to suck back up his own sexual emissions together with those of his partner from her vagina. This was the ultimate way of mingling and consuming sexual fluids as required in early Tantric sex.

Obviously the story about the Dalai Lama was just a fantasy, but what about *vajroli mudra* itself? Is it possible? There are some who claim to be able to do it, including the writers and authorities on Tantra, Dr Jonn Mumford (Swami Anandakapila Saraswati) and André Van Lysebeth. But the religious scholar David Gordon White has his doubts, pointing to research carried out by Richard Darmon in 2002, in which yogis were invited to suck up fluid through a catheter (the standard training method). None succeeded. Nevertheless, it's important to gain control of the relevant muscles and we'll be seeing how to do that in Chapter 8.

Fellatio

Although there are depictions of fellatio in Tantric art, and although the *lingam* was an object of veneration, fellatio never was central to Tantric ritual. As we've seen, authentic Tantric sex was initially about *men* receiving spiritual enlightenment and magical powers through women's sexual fluids, not the other way around. Nevertheless, in modern Tantric sex fellatio is:

▶ *an additional way of giving pleasure*
▶ *a way of extending sex without overusing the* yoni
▶ *fun.*

And there's a surprise. Although little research has been done on the real benefits of women's sexual fluids for men, there's good evidence that men's sexual fluids genuinely *are* beneficial to women (see the factbox, p. 125).

Fellatio is possible in the 69 position, but it puts the woman's tongue on the less sensitive side of the *lingam*, rather than on the frenulum side (underneath) where it can exact the maximum response. Also, as mentioned above, a single-minded focus will normally produce more excitement than mutual pleasuring. The best thing, then, is to alternate between cunnilingus and fellatio, swapping positions so that after the man has lain for a time between his partner's open thighs, she can lay between his open thighs. Other positions for fellatio that put the tongue in the right place are the woman kneeling while the man stands, and the man straddling the woman's breasts while she lies on her back.

Have a go
So you're in position (see above). What now?

▶ **Step 1:** *If your man isn't yet erect, gently circle the underside of the glans (the underside of the reddish-purple tip or head) with a fingertip moistened with saliva. (If your man has a foreskin you'll need to retract it gently to get at the glans.) 'Talking dirty' will speed things up.*
▶ **Step 2:** *Lick the underside of the glans, the frenulum (some people call it the 'string') in the little cleft of the glans, and the area immediately below the string. This will take his erection to a new level.*

- ▶ **Step 3:** *Move to the dark line that runs down the underside of the shaft. When your Shiva's lingam is really hard, this line stands out as a ridge and is then capable of generating some exquisite sensations, if you lick from end to end.*
- ▶ **Step 4:** *Take the head of the lingam into your mouth and continue working on the glans with your tongue.*
- ▶ **Step 5:** *You can now replicate the in-out of vaginal sex, either by moving your head or by letting him thrust (but don't let him thrust too hard or deep). Don't suck the saliva out of your mouth as you suck the lingam. Rather, bathe the lingam in saliva as your tongue glides up and down the glans.*

Tricks
- ▶ *Taking a mouthful of tea just before fellatio can produce a nice warm sensation (and help with lubrication when the mouth is dry).*
- ▶ *Making a little tube of thumb and forefinger just in front of your lips can give him extra sensation when he's thrusting.*
- ▶ *Holding the shaft in your hand can increase stimulation, especially if you also slide it down towards the testicles to tension the skin (but do it very gently).*
- ▶ *Playing with his scrotum and anus during fellatio will take sensation up to a whole new level.*

TIPS FOR SHAKTIS

It's important to realize that a flaccid penis is *not* very sensitive in terms of sexual stimulation. It becomes sensitive as it erects, partly due to the action of oxytocin (see previous chapter) and partly due to the massive increase in blood flow. The only area of the flaccid penis that creates any pleasure at all is the underside of the glans, which is why it's the place to start.

Just as every *yoni* is different, so is every *lingam*. So, if you don't yet know one another very well, encourage your man to guide you with his moans and groans, or ask what feels nice as you go along.

Go easy on the area around and including the opening of the urethra (the hole) – quite a lot of men find it causes pain, not pleasure.

A whitish substance called smegma can build up where the glans of the penis joins the shaft. This is unhealthy for a man and for you too, so don't have sex (oral or vaginal) while smegma is present. The *lingam* needs washing daily, and before a Tantric sex session.

To swallow or not to swallow

Some men like to ejaculate in their lovers' mouths. Some women are excited by this, some don't mind, and some hate the idea. An obvious objection is that once a man has ejaculated he can't have sex again until his refractory period has passed. For some extremely virile young men that might only be a matter of minutes but for most men it will be far longer. That means the woman won't afterwards be able to enjoy vaginal penetration by the *lingam*.

What's the Tantric view? Of course, it's one way for a woman to absorb male sexual fluids but, although it certainly isn't harmful (provided the man has no sexual-health problems), the scientific evidence we have is for the beneficial effects of semen *in the vagina*.

A team led by Gordon Gallup, a psychologist at the State University of New York, looked for a relationship between the sex lives of women and their degree of happiness, using the Beck Depression Inventory (a standard questionnaire for assessing mood). The team discovered that women whose partners never used condoms were significantly happier than women whose partners always or usually used condoms. (The unhappiest were the women who weren't having any sex at all.)

After controlling for various factors, Gallup and his team concluded that the happiest women were, indeed, absorbing 'happy' chemicals from their partner's semen through the walls of their vaginas. This is not very surprising, in fact, because semen contains various mood-altering hormones

(Contd)

including testosterone, oestrogen, follicle-stimulating hormone, luteinizing hormone and various prostaglandins. Several of these chemicals, believed to have come from the man, have been detected in women's bloodstreams soon after sex.

So, from this point of view, should a man ejaculate as much as possible? In reality, a woman will always receive *some* sexual fluid from her partner, and the man who doesn't ejaculate can make up for the smaller quantity by having sex more often.

I must stress that sexually transmitted diseases and unwanted pregnancies would more than offset any of the psychological benefits of semen. So if you need to use condoms then you should continue to do so.

TO SHAVE OR NOT TO SHAVE?

Men who want to enjoy fellatio should, at least, trim their pubic hair so their partners don't get hairs in their mouths. But there's a good argument for going further. Naked skin is far more sensitive than hairy skin. You can prove that for yourself very easily by shaving a small area. So I would suggest that, in addition to a general trim, you should shave the hair on your scrotum. You'll find that when your partner fondles your testicles, especially with lubricant, she'll drive you wild. Don't use a beard trimmer because it may cut the loose skin – your partner's electric shaver will work much better or, nowadays, you too can have a wax.

If your partner is reluctant to perform fellatio the first thing is to make sure it has nothing to do with hygiene. Always wash your *lingam* and the surrounding area before sex (showering together is a good way). If there's still a problem then discuss it in a loving way. Don't be aggressive – a *lingam* can look pretty intimidating.

YOUR WHOLE BODY IS A SEX ORGAN

As part of *nyasa*, the subject of the previous chapter, there's no reason you shouldn't be just as oral with the rest of your partner's body as you are with your partner's genitals. So, spread a little sauce (maybe whipped cream) over your partner's skin and start 'eating' away. Or simply give a 'tongue bath', licking and tasting your partner from head to foot.

10 THINGS TO REMEMBER

1 *Originally, the whole point of Tantric sex was the production of sexual fluids.*

2 *Drinking a woman's sexual fluids (sometimes in combination with a man's) was believed to confer gnosis, or the intuitive understanding of spiritual truths.*

3 *Sexual fluids were also believed to confer* siddhis *or magical powers, such as the power of flight.*

4 *All those who shared the sexual fluids during the* cakrapuja *felt themselves united as a clan or* kula.

5 *Whether we mean to or not, sex usually involves ingesting a certain amount of a partner's bodily fluids.*

6 *The tongue can be far more important in sex than many people realize, being served by five pairs of cranial nerves.*

7 *The 69 position is fun but both cunnilingus and fellatio are usually better when attention is undivided.*

8 *The most sensitive part of the vulva is the clitoris which has 8,000 nerve fibres, twice as many as in the penis.*

9 *The most sensitive part of the penis is the underside of the glans.*

10 *Women can absorb the semen's 'happy' chemicals through the walls of their vaginas.*

HOW TANTRIC ARE YOU NOW?

☐ Have you and your partner shared a 'cocktail' including something from each of your bodies?
☐ Have you sucked and gently bitten your partner's extended tongue?
☐ Has your partner sucked and gently bitten your extended tongue?
☐ Have you passed food and drink from mouth to mouth?
☐ Have you performed oral sex on your partner for at least five minutes?
☐ (Men only) Have you discovered your partner's clitoral glans?
☐ (Men only) Have you given your partner an orgasm from oral sex?
☐ (Women only) Have you taken your partner's *lingam* into your mouth?
☐ (Women only) Have you discovered the most sensitive spot on your partner's *lingam*?
☐ Have you openly discussed oral sex techniques with your partner?
☐ Are you following the tongue exercises?
☐ Have you given your partner a 'tongue bath'?

If you answered 'yes' to between eight and ten questions you're obviously very open to Tantric sex ideas and have worked hard on acquiring the skills.

If you answered 'yes' to between five and seven questions you're on your way but you have quite a bit of experimenting and practising to do.

If you couldn't answer 'yes' to more than four questions, maybe you're thinking that oral sex and sexual fluids are rather, well, primitive? In that case, read the chapter again, mull it over and, perhaps, try out a few ideas on your own. Tantric sex certainly is *earthy* but it's also *heavenly*.

7

Ejaculation – how not to (for him), how to (for her)

In this chapter you will learn:
- *how men can withhold ejaculation*
- *how women can ejaculate*
- *how both can lead to an altered state of consciousness.*

> *Give a hundred thousand loving thrusts to my swollen*
> *three-petalled lotus.*
>
> Chandamaharosana Tantra

Sex without ejaculation is the surest way for a man to reach *and maintain* the mystical state that is the aim of Tantric sex. And, astonishing as it may seem, when a man *doesn't* ejaculate he can both give and receive far, far more pleasure.

The position of women is rather different when it comes to ejaculation. Most aren't aware that they can accomplish something analogous to men, that is, to spurt liquid at the moment of orgasm. A few do it quite naturally, but everyone else has to learn. Women who like to do it say it takes sex up to a whole new level.

So here are two experiences that may be new to you – the man withholding ejaculation and the woman learning *to* ejaculate. Yet both have the same aim of modifying the sexual experience and thereby creating a hugely altered state of consciousness.

Sex without ejaculation

As far as most men are concerned, ejaculation is the whole point of sex. And as far as the average woman is concerned, her partner's ejaculation, timed with one of her own orgasms, is the supreme moment. If her partner didn't ejaculate she'd feel something of a failure, for not having excited him enough. But that's very much a matter of conditioning. And, with a little effort, you can condition yourselves to think, feel and act in a different way.

There are two styles of non-ejaculatory sex for men:

▶ *never closely approaching the 'point of no return' (PNR)*
▶ *so closely approaching the PNR that orgasms are experienced without ejaculation.*

In this chapter we're only going to be looking at the first style, so I'm not going to be explaining here in any detail the distinction between orgasm and ejaculation. We'll be looking at all that in the next chapter, when I'll be describing the second style. For now, just keep in mind that (for both men and women) I'll be using the term 'orgasm' to refer to the highly-pleasurable muscular contractions, 'ejaculation' to mean the emission of fluid and, when it's not clear, 'orgasm/ejaculation' to mean both together.

Getting mystical

Imagine being, as it were, locked together with your lover, *lingam* in *yoni*, resting easily for maybe half an hour, maybe an hour, maybe longer. The air is probably heavy with incense, gentle music is playing and a sort of radiant lethargy has overcome you. Your mind, powered by the 'electricity' of sex, floats freely through beautiful fantasies. Or are they fantasies? Maybe they're not at all. Maybe they're a place beyond *maya*, the 'veil' that obscures the Divine Consciousness from view.

This, for both men and women, is the experience of sex when the man keeps well away from orgasm/ejaculation. It's the kind of sex that's so often pictured in Indian erotic miniatures. There you'll find couples either staring dreamily into one another's eyes or towards some distant realm of intuition, united in the static and sometimes quite complicated poses that provide the 'trance energy'.

Not exciting enough for you? Not really sex at all? But let's analyse it. In the first place, no one is suggesting this should be the style of sex you have all the time, only that it's something you should at least try and, perhaps, enjoy now and then. You could look upon it as half way between an intimate cuddle and full-on sex. Why not? If cuddling is nice, then surely this is even nicer? And when you think about it, it's not *instead of* other sex. It can so easily be *in addition*. In fact, it could be as often as you both like.

Most men can't have sex as frequently as they desire because of the refractory period that follows orgasm/ejaculation. In some young men this may only be a matter of minutes, but in older men it can be a matter of hours or even days. What's more, the average man tends to lose interest once he's ejaculated, so there's little chance of more *auparishtaka* either. In other words, a woman who doesn't have an orgasm before her partner ejaculates is unlikely to have one afterwards. But if there's no ejaculation there's no refractory period.

And if there's no ejaculation, sex can also be as long as you like. As noted in Chapter 1, Kinsey concluded that in 1940s America intercourse generally lasted a pitiful two minutes – that's to say, for three-quarters of men, ejaculation occurred within two minutes of entering the vagina. Nowadays, surveys suggest the norm is from six to ten minutes. But without ejaculation, *hours* of pleasure become possible.

Of course, this style of Tantric sex isn't about setting endurance records. It isn't time for its own sake. Rather, it's a kind of meditation. A highly spiritual experience. That happy sense of oneness with your partner (or even the cosmos) is best realized not in the brief heat of orgasm/ejaculation but in the gentle pond of reflection.

So, in fact, there's quite a lot going for this. When a man keeps well away from orgasm/ejaculation:

▶ *you can focus on your spiritual goals (the whole point of genuine Tantric sex) in a sex-induced altered state of consciousness.*
▶ *you can both enjoy a different kind of quiet but profound intimacy, even if you're not especially interested in spiritual things*
▶ *you (the man) never develop a 'sexual hangover' in which, because of hormonal changes, you lose desire for your partner (see below)*
▶ *you (the woman) never experience that post-coital let-down in which your partner rolls over, ignores you and goes to sleep*
▶ *you can have sex as long as you want*
▶ *you can have sex again as soon as you both want.*

The sexual hangover

In India it was believed that semen was the physical embodiment of a kind of energy known in Sanskrit as **bindu**. Men who conserved their *bindu* would become full of *tejas* (radiant energy). This is an idea that goes back a long way. According to the *Brihadaranyaka Upanishad*, one of the very earliest *Upanishads* and therefore written down almost three thousand years ago, a man who has ejaculated should rub the semen between his breasts or eyebrows, saying: 'Let the semen return to me, let vigour come to me again, let glow and good fortune come to me again.'

Frequent ejaculation does cause men to feel 'hung over', especially as they get older. When a man ejaculates he depletes his store of mature sperm, each one of which has taken 70 days to create. So sperm are not in inexhaustible supply. However, it's not sperm that are really the issue (they make up only a small percentage of the semen, ranging from about one per cent of the volume up to about ten per cent, depending on the individual, the frequency of ejaculation and the particular scientific study). The real issue is prolactin, a chemical secreted by the pituitary gland following ejaculation (or stress or extremely vigorous exercise). Prolactin decreases sex drive, decreases testosterone and, in sufficient quantity, can actually cause impotence. Ejaculation can also negatively impact the 'happy' neurotransmitter systems involving serotonin and dopamine. The effects of all this can last several days.

It's a simple 'trick' of evolution. The human race wouldn't survive without sex but nor would it if men and women had sex all the time. When a man ejaculates too much (relative to virility) the prolactin reaches a level at which he physically can't have any more sex with you. Our male ancestors, after sex, were thus freed to search for mammoths and so on.

Here's the cunning bit. If a man encounters a *different* woman his hormones change and he's capable of sex once more. You see, from an evolutionary perspective there was no point in having more sex with *you* because you might already be pregnant. The best strategy for a man to perpetuate his 'selfish genes' is to have sex with a *new woman*. That's the 'sexual hangover'. You seem less attractive, other women seem more attractive – and if there are no other women, the man is just plain irritable.

Women, too, can experience a sexual 'hangover'. But in their case they produce prolactin not only at orgasm but also during intercourse. So there seems to be no comparable way for women to avoid it. Fortunately, a woman's 'hangover' seems to be much less pronounced.

As far as men are concerned, the extent of a sexual hangover depends on the frequency of ejaculation. However, there's no set number of ejaculations per week that's right for everybody. We're all different. If ejaculation makes you feel elated and happy afterwards then you're not ejaculating too much. But if you feel flat as soon as you've ejaculated then you're ejaculating too often. The intriguing ability of a man to overcome the refractory period should a new partner come along is known as the Coolidge effect. The story is that the 30th American president Calvin Coolidge was visiting a farm with his wife. After watching the chickens for a while Mrs Coolidge asked the farmer how often the cock had sex. 'Several times a day,' came the reply. She nudged the farmer and said, 'Tell that to the president.' Mr Coolidge then asked, 'Always the same chicken?' 'Nope,' replied the farmer. 'Different chicken every time.' The president nudged the farmer. 'Tell that to Mrs Coolidge,' he said.

The Coolidge effect proves that men can overcome the 'hangover' when they treat their partners as goddesses and realize that they have many different aspects. Today, you make love to one woman, tomorrow you make love to a 'different' woman. And the same applies to women when they treat their partners as gods. There's so much to discover about one another.

The authentic traditions

Given that the production of sexual fluids was central to early Tantric sex ritual, how did it come about that men withholding ejaculation should be seen as the key to Tantric sex in the twenty-first century? Is it really part of authentic Tantric sex at all?

In fact, deferring or withholding ejaculation wasn't specifically Tantric. In a certain era it was the practice of all Hindus, as the explorer and sexologist Sir Richard Burton made clear in his commentary to the Indian sex manual, the *Ananga Ranga* (Stage of Love), when it was published in English in 1885:

> *The reader will bear in mind that the exceeding pliability*
> *of the Hindu's limbs enables him to assume attitudes*
> *absolutely impossible to the European, and his chief object*
> *in congress is to avoid tension of the muscles, which would*

*shorten the period of enjoyment. For which reason, even in
the act of love, he will delay to talk, to caress his wife, to
eat, to drink, chew Pan-supari [betel], and perhaps smoke a
waterpipe.*

Some erotic Indian miniatures even show women playing musical
instruments and men practising archery during lovemaking. All this
may seem quite comical to Westerners but these are the kinds of
things we'll be trying out in this chapter. And you'll probably find
you enjoy them quite a lot.

Most likely the idea originated not in India but among the Chinese
Taoists. The Taoist philosophy of living in harmony with the forces
of nature goes back at least two and a half thousand years, long
before formal Tantra. In sexual terms, it means making love in
a way which recognizes that men are yang (quick to arouse and,
like fire, burning fiercely) and that women are yin (slow to arouse
but ultimately, like water, more powerful). In other words, a man
needed to develop the skill of slow combustion using, as many
early Taoist texts advised, 'a thousand loving thrusts'.

This was considered so important that the seventh century *T'ung
Hsüan Tzu* devoted seven chapters to the various ways those
thrusts can be made. That India was influenced by this seems
clear from the *Chandamaharosana Tantra* in which the goddess
Vajrayogini invites the Tantrika to survey her 'three-petalled lotus'
(the two inner labia and the hood of the clitoris) and to penetrate
it with a 'fully awakened sceptre' moving 'a hundred thousand
times'. What was specific to Tantric sex was the appropriation of
the altered state of consciousness for spiritual ends.

The Tantras are mostly silent on specific ways of having sex
without orgasm/ejaculation. That kind of practical information
seems to have been passed on mostly by gurus in person and was
(and is) kept secret by initiates. One of the few written clues in
Tantric texts comes from the sixteenth century *Kaulavalinirnaya*
which says a man should chew betel, unite *lingam* and *yoni*,
and worship the woman 'with the pleasures of love' until she's

'agitated' (that's to say, anxious for orgasm) while calmly repeating his mantra 1008 times followed by another 108 times. So mantras were used for ejaculation control by focusing the mind on spiritual matters (turn back to Chapter 4 if you've forgotten about them).

We do have a nineteenth century description of Tantric ritual involving this kind of sex. In a book called *L'Inde que j'ai connue* (The India I Knew), published in Paris in 1951, Alexandra David-Néel recounts how she spied on a Tantric ceremony. After the usual lengthy preliminaries she saw each man pull his Shakti against him for ritualistic intercourse which she described as 'perfectly chaste'. The key point is that the worshippers then remained as motionless as 'the sculptures of Hindu gods embracing their goddesses'. To her it was a religious act 'devoid of any obscenities'.

Swami Muktananda

Swami Muktananda (1908–82), known as Baba, was almost certainly one of the most recent links in an unbroken chain of oral transmission. He concealed his techniques, even from many of his followers, behind a façade of celibacy. But his method of giving Shaktipat (that is, the transmission of Shakti or the power of the goddess) was sexual, at least at times. Lis Harris, a journalist writing for the New Yorker, tracked down one female ex-devotee who described an incident that occurred when she was 26 and Baba was 71. Apparently, Baba had explained to her that 'when *Kundalini* is fully realized the body exists in a state of permanent ecstasy'. He then asked her to lie on a table and, according to her account, 'placed himself inside of me' and they stayed like that for about 90 minutes during which Baba was said not to have ejaculated, nor even to have had an erection, nor moved. They just talked. Nevertheless, the woman described it as 'a very extraordinary experience' which created in her 'a state of total ecstasy'. Although she said it had 'nothing

(Contd)

to do with sex' it's clear it *was* a style of Tantric sex, lengthy and without ejaculation, designed to awaken *Kundalini* in her.

Whether or not you want to learn from a guru is up to you but, personally, I wouldn't recommend you swap what is one of your most precious treasures, that is, free will, for a lesson in sex. Not even Tantric sex.

Have a go
▶ **Step 1:** *Agree that you will have (and compare) two sex sessions in which you, the man, don't experience orgasm/ ejaculation. You, the woman, will have an orgasm or orgasms in one of the sessions, but no orgasms at all in the other.*
▶ **Step 2:** *Choose times when you're both feeling tranquil and create a beautiful, spiritual atmosphere with (for example) nice furnishings, candles, incense, music, jewellery and, above all, beautiful thoughts.*
▶ **Step 3:** *Arouse yourselves with* nyasa *(Chapter 5) and* auparishtaka *(Chapter 6), but without the man getting anywhere near orgasm/ejaculation.*
▶ **Step 4:** *In a very, very comfortable place, unite yoni and lingam in one of the more static postures such as* yab yum *or* mula bandha *(see Chapter 10).*
▶ **Step 5:** *Don't move more than is necessary to create a sexual current. You, the man, will probably want to maintain an erection but, in fact, in* mula bandha *it's perfectly possible to remain inside your partner even if your erection subsides. You, the woman, will forego orgasm in one session but in the other you should enjoy one or more orgasms by clitoral stimulation. Both think beautiful thoughts for an hour – more, if you wish. Nice music will help. You could stare into one another's eyes, co-ordinate breathing and reflect on how much you love one-another. Or you could aim for a more transcendent experience in which you meditate on your connection with the entire universe. In particular, focus on* Kundalini *(see Chapter 2) and*

visualize the sexual energy gradually moving up your spine and into your brain.

▶ **Step 6:** *There is nothing that naturally brings this kind of Tantric sex to an end. Just stop when you both feel like it – but a proper trial needs at least an hour per session.*

▶ **Step 7:** *Discuss the two different sessions. Did either of them create, in either of you, a significantly altered state of consciousness? Did you feel as if the boundaries between your physical bodies had lifted? Did you feel merged into one another? Did you feel part of the 'great oneness'. If so, great. If not, it's still a very pleasant way of relaxing intimately together for a while.*

HOW IT FEELS TO A WOMAN

When Shiva keeps well away from orgasm/ejaculation, you, Shakti, have two options. Either you, too, can remain in what the sex researchers Masters and Johnson called the 'plateau phase' – that's to say, between the initial 'excitement phase' and the 'orgasmic phase'. Or you can have orgasms by whatever means you like.

Most women very easily remain at the plateau level. As Masters and Johnson showed, the resolution phase (when things return to normal) is then considerably extended as a sensual and very enjoyable 'afterglow'. But how enjoyable is the plateau phase? In my focus groups many women say there would be no point in sex without orgasm (something that runs contrary to the way women are 'supposed' to be). On the other hand, the sex researcher Shere Hite heard from women who masturbated as much as two or three times a day even though they never had orgasms – clear proof that some women find sex without orgasm perfectly pleasurable.

The Tantras themselves give little insight into how different sexual techniques were supposed to feel and almost nothing in them was written from the woman's viewpoint. However, we do have a Victorian account of sorts, written by a remarkable American doctor by the name of Alice Bunker Stockham. Born in 1833, Stockham visited India and was inspired to develop her own

version of Tantric sex, which she described in her book
Karezza – Ethics of Marriage (1903). A couple should begin, she
wrote, with a period of meditation 'to allow free usurpation of
cosmic intelligence'. Then, 'with expressions of endearment and
affection' came 'the complete but quiet union of the sexual organs'.
Orgasm/ejaculation was avoided not by any Western form of *japa*
but simply by never getting very excited:

> *During a lengthy period of perfect control the whole being of
> each is submerged into the other, and an exquisite exaltation
> experienced. This may be followed by a quiet motion…
> In the course of an hour the physical tension subsides, the
> spiritual exaltation increases, and not uncommonly visions
> of a transcendent life are seen and consciousness of new
> powers experienced.*

Karezza, then, was spiritual sex. But the mindset was very different
to Tantra. In *Karezza*, Stockham wrote, 'there is no defilement
or debasement in the natural and controlled expression of sexual
love'. Authentic Tantrikas, by contrast, were prepared to go to
almost any length in pursuit of 'spiritual sex' and often considered
'defilement' as an essential part of it. Nevertheless, Stockham wrote
a beautiful description of the altered state of consciousness that
was the aim of both Tantric sex and Karezza. Sex, she wrote, 'must
be experienced upon a higher plane than the merely physical.'

And what if you want orgasms? Unless your man is skilled in the
techniques described in the next chapter he won't be able to give
them to you using his *lingam*. But there are other means, the most
powerful being that, while *lingam* and *yoni* are united, either of
you gives the *yonimani* some attention with a finger.

Insight

Some schools of Tantra believe that since women don't
ejaculate like men and therefore, it's argued, expend nothing
(but see Ejaculation for women, p. 142) they can have as
many orgasms as they like during this kind of sex. Others
argue that if non-orgasm/ejaculation brings spiritual benefits

to men, then women should have access to the same benefits, also through non-orgasm/ejaculation. In my focus groups, some women did report that non-orgasm/ejaculation brought a wonderful 'glow' but others said it brought frustration. That seems to be linked to both the mental approach and the degree of arousal (see the factbox below).

HOW IT FEELS TO A MAN

A century before Masters and Johnson, the founder of the 'free love' Oneida Community in New York wrote his own colourful description of the phases of arousal. To John Humphrey Noyes, sex for a man was like a 'stream in three conditions':

▶ *still water above rapids*
▶ *a course of rapids above a waterfall*
▶ *a waterfall.*

Noyes recommended remaining in 'the region of easy rowing'. That's to say, a man could approach orgasm/ejaculation, but never so closely as to risk 'going over' the falls. His motive, however, wasn't so much spiritual as to keep down the rate of pregnancy. A vulcanized rubber condom had gone into production four years earlier but it was about as thick as a pair of rubber gloves. Noyes' method was clearly far more popular because community members reportedly had an average of about three partners a week.

Remaining in calm waters needs no special skill but in the next chapter we'll be learning the very special techniques that will allow you to go to the very top of the waterfall *and stay there.*

Arousal and frustration

This is a style of sex that should result in a combination of sensual and spiritual radiance. Some men and women,

(Contd)

however, find it results in frustration. The key seems to be in the expectation and in the degree of arousal. This is not to be looked upon as a sort of second-rate intercourse but as a particular style of sex in its own right with its own very special qualities. In women, vasocongestion in the pelvic organs (that's to say, the build-up of blood) can become uncomfortable and even painful if not relieved by orgasm. That leaves women feeling irritable, not mystical. Either the woman needs to have orgasms or the degree of arousal has to be kept to a sort of intense cuddling with just enough stimulation for the *yoni* to be receptive. Men may initially find it helps to look upon the whole thing as a challenge to their powers of self-control, with non-ejaculation thus becoming a source of satisfaction rather than frustration.

Ejaculation for women

It's quite possible that many women ejaculate to a limited extent without even knowing it. But when women ejaculate on purpose or, at least, knowingly, it adds a thrilling dimension to sex, physically, emotionally and spiritually. Women who do it find it takes sex to a whole new level. The excitement can be extreme. In addition to this 'hidden' ejaculation, every woman can perform at least one of the two main forms of 'squirting' – it's simply a question of overcoming inhibitions.

As for their partners, some don't like being squirted on but others like it a lot. If you enjoy getting wet, if you find the idea of being drenched by your partner's sexual fluids intimate and arousing then you'll be an enthusiastic accomplice.

But what exactly is **female ejaculation** and was it ever an authentic part of traditional Tantric sex?

WHAT IS FEMALE EJACULATION?

Sexologists are still arguing over female ejaculation. Some say
the liquid comes from the female equivalent of the male prostate,
known as 'Skene's glands' or the 'female prostate'. Others say it
comes from the bladder – in other words, it's urine.

In reality it really doesn't matter. Where the liquid comes from is a
side issue (but one we'll nevertheless settle in a moment). There are
more important questions. Such as, is it exciting? Is it thrilling? Can
it blow your mind (that is, help you into an altered Tantric state of
consciousness)? More and more women are saying yes, yes, yes.

Possibly you're now thinking that if it *is* urine you don't want
anything to do with it. Why would you want to pee yourself
during sex? Why would your partner want you to? But that way
of thinking is all down to conditioning. After all, what makes you
think the liquid in the Skene's glands is 'nicer' than pee, anyway?
In fact, there's nothing the matter with a healthy person's urine.
In the East, urine has long been used medicinally and *amaroli* or
'urine therapy' has its followers in the West too.

To my knowledge, there's no scientific evidence that drinking
your own urine is beneficial, beyond the possibility that the
high melatonin content of first morning urine *might* promote
meditation. But nor is there any evidence that getting splashed
with urine is any more harmful than getting splashed by vaginal
secretions, semen or the contents of the female prostate.

Remember that it's part of Tantric sex to break taboos. So why not
tackle the taboo over urine?

All right, so is it urine or is it something else? Well, it's...

- ▶ sometimes *fluid from the female prostate*
- ▶ sometimes *urine*
- ▶ sometimes *a mixture of the two*.

I'm not going to say that one form of ejaculation is any more genuine than another. When the quantity of liquid is small (say, less than a teaspoonful) then it's probably from the female prostate. When the quantity is large (possibly as much as a cupful) then it's either entirely from the bladder or a mixture of bladder and female prostate. The bladder just has to be involved because the female prostate is smaller than the male's and there's absolutely no way it could generate and store so much liquid in the time. But that's not really the issue. The issue is how it *feels*. So here's why you should at least try both main forms of female ejaculation:

▶ *You may achieve an extremely altered state of consciousness, which is the aim of Tantric sex.*
▶ *Tantric sex is all about expanding horizons, being open to new ideas and overturning taboos.*
▶ *Many women report that ejaculating provides an emotional release that surpasses 'normal' sex.*
▶ *Variety is important if you're going to enjoy a long sex life (especially with the same person).*
▶ *It can be enormously exciting for both you and your partner.*

HOW FEMALE EJACULATION WORKS

So, in fact, there are two mechanisms involved, one for the bladder and one for the female prostate.

The bladder (in women) is surrounded by the vagina, the uterus and the pubic bone. When a woman has an orgasm, if it's a big one, then both the vagina *and* the uterus go into spasms, compressing the bladder against the bone. Normally, the bladder sphincter prevents any urine escaping, but if the sphincter is relaxed (by stimulation of the G-spot, as we'll see in a moment) then the violent movements of the vagina and uterus fire some of the urine out of the urethra (which, of course, opens into the entrance to the vagina). The distance can be considerable.

The female prostate, like the bladder, is connected to the urethra, which means that whatever the source of the fluid it all comes out of the same place – you can't tell the source of the liquid simply by looking. It's aligned with the slightly raised, corrugated area on the front wall of the vagina that's known as the G-spot. Stimulating the G-spot inside the vagina therefore stimulates the female prostate, which is located on the other side of the vaginal wall. At the same time it causes the bladder sphincter to relax and open.

Women emit fluid from their prostate glands often. Prostate-specific acid phosphatase (PSAP or PAP) is one of the things that can leave a mark on underwear. So, in all probability, most women also emit fluid from their prostate glands during sex. In that case, why don't they know and why don't their partners know? In the first place, the quantity can be so small that it goes unnoticed. Secondly, it seems women may register the trickle of fluid as an escape of urine and clamp down, thus causing a retrograde and therefore invisible ejaculation into the bladder. Whatever the explanation, what we need to do, rather than just let it seep out, is find a way to squirt it.

A GUIDE TO SQUIRTING

Women who 'squirt' during sex or masturbation experience a whole new thrilling dimension. They may alter their states of consciousness far more than they otherwise would, thus achieving through ejaculation the same mind-effects that men (paradoxically) can achieve by not ejaculating. As for the men, many see it as like being initiated into a great mystery, as becoming an even more intimate part of their partners' lives.

The following method is in two stages. Initially, you're going to learn to ejaculate urine (not the same thing as urination) simultaneously with orgasm. Once you've mastered that, you're going to *try* to learn to ejaculate from your prostate (it's not clear whether or not all women can achieve this particular kind of ejaculation). That's the easiest order to learn and it doesn't mean ejaculating from the prostate is somehow 'better' or 'more advanced'. If you acquire both skills you can choose to ejaculate urine or ejaculate prostatic fluid as you wish.

Have a go – ejaculating urine

Remember this is all about squirting a burst of urine under enormous pressure, not emptying the entire contents of your bladder in the usual way.

▶ Step 1: *Drink a couple of glasses of water. Think about what you're going to do. Get relaxed about it. Visualize it. (If you're having a problem with the whole idea of squirting urine, the Betty Erickson self-hypnosis method, described in the next chapter, may help.)*

▶ Step 2: *Find a place you feel safe and comfortable masturbating and that you don't mind getting wet. Some sexologists suggest practising in the bath but, in my experience, most women are put off by that. The bed is fine but you'll probably want to protect it with a couple of large, thick towels.*

▶ Step 3: *Self-stimulate in your usual way. Once things are going well, focus attention on your G-spot, either with one or two fingers or with a dildo – the elegant, glass models are great for this. (If you're not familiar with your G-spot take a look at the section opposite.) A lubricant will help and is pretty much essential for older women. Experiment with different pressures, strokes and places – some women find there's a particular part of the G-spot that's especially good. Teasing your clitoris may help build the orgasmic momentum and also overcome the G-spot discomfort that some women experience before the pleasurable sensations take over.*

▶ Step 4: *Let the urge to orgasm and the desire to release urine build up towards a simultaneous peak. You need to get to the point where you feel you just can't hold back the contents of your bladder any longer. Then go for the orgasm. At the very point of orgasm remove the dildo (or finger) and press out. Try to squirt a jet rather than release the whole lot. Some women find it helps to deliberately cry out ('Yes, yes, yesssss!') but that will probably come automatically.*

▶ Step 5: *If it worked and you didn't empty your whole bladder you'll have enough to do it again if you want. You may find you can 'squirt' several times in a session. If it didn't work, keep on trying.*

Have a go – ejaculating prostatic fluid

Once you've perfected and enjoyed the technique of squirting urine over several sessions you might like to move on to deliberately ejaculating from the prostate. The method is very similar.

▶ **Step 1:** *Empty your bladder. Don't have anything to drink.*

▶ **Step 2:** *As before, find a place you feel safe and comfortable masturbating. This time there won't be much liquid but you still might like to protect bedding or furnishings with a towel.*

▶ **Step 3:** *Self-stimulate in your usual way and once things are going well focus attention on your G-spot. You'll know from your earlier adventures in ejaculation exactly how and where to apply the pressure. Don't forget the lubricant, especially if you're an older women.*

▶ **Step 4:** *When orgasm occurs, remove the dildo (or finger), relax your bladder and press out as if urinating, even though this time your bladder is more or less empty.*

▶ **Step 5:** *If it worked you should have felt a new and stronger sensation, although you may not actually have noticed the extra liquid at the time – the quantity that comes from the prostate is very small. If it didn't work, keep trying. If you can't make it work for you after a few tries, don't worry. The orgasm should be pretty good anyway, and it may be the case that it's anatomically impossible for you to 'fire' prostatic fluid – the jury is out on how many women can and can't. You can still ejaculate urine when you want and that's just as exciting, possibly more so.*

The G-spot

Some sexologists are still arguing that the G-spot, named after the German researcher Ernst Gräfenberg, doesn't exist. Well, it does. It may or may not give you a great deal of pleasure, but that's a completely different issue. The G-spot is located on the front wall of the vagina and, in the majority of women, it's just inside the entrance and about the size of a fingernail. In other words, if you lie on your back and push a finger through the resistance of the opening, pad upwards, the very next thing you'll feel on the roof of your vagina is the G-spot. In a small proportion of women it's slightly further back. Wherever yours is, you'll know it at once because it will feel slightly rougher than the rest of the vagina. If you can't identify it, wait until you're really excited. At that stage the roughness will become so accentuated that the area feels corrugated.

Behind the G-spot, on the other side of the vaginal wall, lie the urethra and the female prostate. So when you stimulate your G-spot, you're stimulating your prostate as well as your urethra – which is why it makes you feel as if you want to urinate.

Unlike the clitoris, the G-spot is far less predictable. Some women love G-spot stimulation from the moment they discover it, some grow to like it more and more, and some never get to enjoy it at all. Part of the problem is that the initial feelings, before the pleasure takes over, *can* seem unpleasant and even painful. So experimenting with your G-spot requires a little faith. In my focus groups, G-spot experience is quite varied. Some women say they never feel any discomfort, others (usually older women) say they experience stinging and even pain. Some women say they need a great deal of stimulation, others that they need *less* than for the clitoris. Every body is different.

Squirting with a partner

It may be it was you, the woman, who took the initiative over learning to ejaculate. Or it may have been your partner. If it was you, you may have to convince your partner. Some men love the idea and, at the time of writing, it's the top search topic on several porn sites. Others don't appreciate it at all. So you may have to explain your feelings and you'll almost certainly have to explain the methods. Even if your partner understands the general idea you'll still have to guide him to the exact spot and let him know what movements to use and how much pressure to apply.

If your partner is going to use a dildo then you'll probably just lie on your back. But if you're going to try to ejaculate during intercourse then there are some special considerations. The standard missionary doesn't bring the penis into very strong contact with the G-spot. A solution to that is to raise your hips on a couple of pillows so your partner's thrusting will be upwards. Better are the rear-entry positions (see Chapter 10) which make it easier for your partner to get the right alignment. Try lying face down with a pillow under your hips and your partner sitting on the backs of your thighs. It's a position that almost automatically ensures not only the perfect trajectory but also the perfect depth. If you can ejaculate with a dildo but not with a *lingam*, then try a standing up position – a lot of women report that, although it's not the most comfortable way, it's the one in which it's easiest to ejaculate. Whatever position you use, remind your partner to keep his *lingam* on the area of the G-spot and not to thrust too deeply.

You may need to discuss what you'll do if things get uncomfortable or even slightly painful before they get exciting. That is certainly the experience of some women. The decision to stop or to go on has to be up to you, based on your knowledge of your own body when masturbating.

TIPS FOR MEN

Men, learn to love getting wet. This is vitally important because if your lover is made to feel at all embarrassed then she'll be inhibited and it just won't happen. Don't say to your lover that you 'don't mind'. That isn't good enough. Convince her how much you would love to be part of such a thrilling and intimate experience.

If you don't know anything about your lover's G-spot, the first thing to do is explore it with the tip of a lubricated forefinger (nail well trimmed) – for how to find it see the text on p. 147. Be very gentle at first. Just tickle it with a 'come here' motion. The less pressure you have to use, the less your partner will feel sore afterwards, and the more often she'll want to do it. Ask your partner to tell you where feels best. If she doesn't get excited straight away, don't take that as a sign you need to increase the stimulation. You may just need to take more time to allow the feelings to build up.

When using your *lingam*, remember that the G-spot is only a little way inside the *yoni* in most women, so there's no point thrusting away down to the cervix. You need to aim the head of your *lingam* quite specifically at the target. If you hold the shaft of in your hand you'll be able to be more precise.

CAN MEN EJACULATE URINE?

It's not generally realized that men can accomplish something similar to a woman's ejaculation of urine. If you're a man who would like to have some idea of what it feels like to a woman, here's how.

- ▶ Step 1: *Wait until you have an urgent desire to urinate.*
- ▶ Step 2: *Masturbate until you have a strong erection and are very close to ejaculating.*
- ▶ Step 3: *Allow your erection to subside just sufficiently to be able to urinate.*
- ▶ Step 4: *Release the urine in short, orgasmic bursts by contracting and relaxing the sphincter as in* vajroli mudra.

Unlike women, men can't actually orgasm and ejaculate urine at the same time and the resulting sensations are therefore less intense but, nevertheless, highly pleasurable.

A FINAL WORD ON FEMALE EJACULATION

Urine was one of the 'five nectars' of Tantra. The others were saliva, menstrual blood, sexual fluids (women's and men's) and excrement. Used ritualistically, these were believed to have magical powers. Nowadays, rational people don't believe in magic but, as we've seen, there are other Tantric reasons for practising female ejaculation, particularly the more powerfully altered state of consciousness that may be possible. But if you don't enjoy ejaculating (or just can't seem to do it) that doesn't make your lovemaking any less Tantric.

10 THINGS TO REMEMBER

1 When a man intentionally keeps well away from the 'point of no return' (PNR), neither experiencing orgasm nor ejaculation, lengthy, meditative sex sessions become possible – with plenty of time to rouse Kundalini.

2 During these long sessions a woman may also forego orgasm, thus experiencing the same kind of mental state as her partner, or she may choose to enjoy orgasms by clitoral stimulation.

3 A man who doesn't ejaculate during sex avoids the possibility of the 'sexual hangover' in which chemical reactions in the body can cause loss of desire and irritability.

4 When a man doesn't ejaculate, a couple can have as much sex as they want.

5 All women can learn to ejaculate a burst of urine; it's not clear what proportion of women can also learn to ejaculate from the female prostate, also known as Skene's glands.

6 Female ejaculation can create intense excitement and emotional release.

7 Female ejaculation is induced by stimulation of the G-spot with a pushing-out at the moment of orgasm.

8 The G-spot does exist. It's the rougher area of skin just inside the entrance to the vagina on the front wall. On the other side of the wall lie the urethra and the female prostate.

9 Some men love getting soaked by their partners' ejaculations; others will need convincing.

10 In authentic, traditional Tantric sex, men used women; in modern Tantric sex women and men are equal.

HOW TANTRIC ARE YOU NOW (MEN)?

- ☐ Have you experimented with hour-long intercourse without experiencing either orgasm or ejaculation?
- ☐ Did these long sessions enable you to create an altered state of consciousness?
- ☐ Were you able to use that altered state of consciousness to explore your spiritual feelings?
- ☐ Have you located and stimulated your partner's G-spot?
- ☐ Have you helped your partner to squirt, either using a dildo or your fingers?
- ☐ Have you enjoyed being soaked by your partner's sexual fluids, either when masturbating her or during intercourse?

If you answered 'yes' to between four and six questions you (and your partner) are obviously very open to Tantric sex ideas and techniques.

If you answered 'yes' to two or three questions you're on your way but you have quite a bit of experimenting to do. There's no rush. Certainly don't put pressure on your partner if she's reluctant – you have years ahead of you to experiment with these things. It will happen when the time is right.

If you couldn't answer 'yes' to more than one question, read the chapter again, together with your partner, and discuss the ideas in an open and easy-going manner. Afterwards, leave time – a few weeks – for a period of reflection. Neither of you should feel you're being forced into doing something you don't want to do. Just enjoy the things you do like together.

HOW TANTRIC ARE YOU
NOW (WOMEN)?

☐ Have you experimented with both orgasmic and non-orgasmic sessions, while your partner kept well away from the 'point of no return' (PNR)?
☐ Did these long sessions enable you to create an altered state of consciousness?
☐ Were you able to use that altered state of consciousness to explore your spiritual feelings?
☐ Have you located and stimulated your G-spot?
☐ Have you been able to squirt urine during private masturbation sessions?
☐ Have you been able to squirt prostatic fluid during private masturbation sessions?
☐ Have you overcome any inhibitions you may have had about squirting during sex with your partner?

If you answered 'yes' to between four and seven questions you (and your partner) are obviously very open to Tantric sex ideas and techniques.

If you answered 'yes' to two or three questions you're on your way but you have quite a bit of experimenting to do. There's no rush. It will happen when the time is right.

If you couldn't answer 'yes' to more than one question, read the chapter again, together with your partner, and discuss the ideas in an open and easy-going manner. Afterwards, leave time – a few weeks – for a period of reflection. Neither of you should feel you're being forced into doing something you don't want to do. Just enjoy the things you do like together.

8

Multiple and simultaneous orgasms

In this chapter you will learn:
- *how men can experience multiple orgasms*
- *how women can experience multiple orgasms*
- *how you can enjoy simultaneous orgasms every time.*

He is a hero who has controlled his senses.

Tantric saying

Imagine that you've been making love for an hour. By now your brain is pumped so full of 'happy chemicals' that you're in a state of bliss that will take hours to fade. You have no idea where your body begins and ends, which bits are yours and which your partner's. Your vision has closed in so much you can hardly see anything except the tangle of limbs. A new touch on almost any part of your body sends something like an electric shock right through you. Your brain is greedy for more and more chemicals by no matter what means. You've lost all sense of inhibition. Taboos have been swept away. You've had so many orgasms you've lost count. Your partner feels the same. But here's the extraordinary thing: you are a *man*. You, a man, are enjoying orgasm after orgasm, just as your partner is.

Male multiple orgasms are popularly believed to be the defining technique of Tantric sex. In fact, they're not. As we've seen,

Tantric sex is all about using sexual energy to create a very special altered state of consciousness. Various techniques can achieve that goal. But – and this is the key point – when you, the man, can experience multiple orgasms then you *both* have the surest and fastest path to that special state of rapture which is the Tantric experience, because when a man has developed sufficient control to enjoy multiple orgasms, so his partner also has the time to enjoy multiple orgasms. And a final simultaneous orgasm is – if you choose – absolutely guaranteed.

Multiple orgasms for men

Normally the man is the limiting factor in sex. For most men, according to surveys, intercourse ends within ten minutes in a single ejaculation. That gives women very little time to revel in their own *natural* multi-orgasmic capacity. And, when sex lasts only a few minutes, neither can reach the state of ecstasy that is the aim of Tantric sex.

There are three possible ways of extending intercourse. One, dealt with in the previous chapter, involves keeping well away from orgasm/ejaculation. That produces a gentle and potentially luminous style of sex. But it's not the erotic, passionate kind of sex that most of us want most of the time. The other two possibilities are:

▶ *training the body to be able to experience orgasm/ejaculation several times in succession*
▶ *training the body to be able to orgasm without ejaculation.*

EJACULATORY VERSUS NON-EJACULATORY ORGASMS

Back in 1995, the sex researchers at Rutgers University, New Jersey, were very excited. They had in front of them a 35-year-old man who was *naturally* capable of multiple ejaculatory orgasms. We're not talking of, say, three or four in a whole night of sex.

This man, without employing any special techniques, was able to self-stimulate to six ejaculations in just 36 minutes, as he proceeded to demonstrate under laboratory conditions.

How did he do it? It had something to do with the amount of semen. His first ejaculation produced around 2.5ml while each of the subsequent ejaculations produced a mere 0.5ml or less. That means the total of his six ejaculations was little more than the average single ejaculation of the average man.

In India, a few years earlier, Dr Prakash Kothari had also studied a man capable of six ejaculations in quick succession under laboratory conditions. But in this case the 30-year-old subject employed *artificial* means. Through exercise he had strengthened his pubococcygeus (PC) muscle (see p. 27) so as to be able to restrict the emission of semen once ejaculation had been triggered. The volume of his ejaculations was also very revealing. One was negligible, one was 1.2 ml, and the rest were in between. Again, the total was only roughly equivalent to one single ejaculation by an average man.

The (not surprising) conclusion is that in order to experience multiple ejaculatory orgasms, the volume of semen needs to be limited in some way. The problem is this: *All the artificial methods of limiting ejaculation, once it has begun, significantly reduce pleasure.*

What's more, some are difficult to learn, others are potentially harmful and, for all of them there's still an eventual limit to the number of ejaculations that are possible. I'll be explaining a little more about them as the chapter progresses but I won't be recommending them. Instead I'll be showing you how you can achieve everything you want very simply and without any risk. Rather than strangling the ejaculation once it's started, you'll learn how to orgasm *without* ejaculation. Here are the advantages:

▶ *virtually unlimited orgasms since hardly any semen is emitted*
▶ *intercourse for an hour or even several hours becomes possible*

- no interference with the pleasure created by each non-ejaculatory orgasm
- no interference with the rhythm of lovemaking
- you can both build a state of excitement far higher than in 'normal' sex
- you readily enter a mystical state in which the boundaries between you and your partner (and possibly the entire universe) seem to break down – which is the aim of Tantric sex
- you maintain a constant state of desire for your partner
- you can have sex again very soon
- the techniques are quick and easy to learn
- there's no risk of any damage to the sexual apparatus.

HOW IT FEELS TO A MAN

What does orgasm without ejaculation feel like? It feels amazing. If I had to choose between only ever being able to have orgasm with ejaculation or orgasm without ejaculation then I'd choose the non-ejaculatory route without hesitation. No kind of sex I've had has ever produced in me such a state of ecstatic, blissful radiance. It becomes a kind of 'brain orgasm' in which the focus shifts from the genitals to the place it matters most of all, the mind. Isn't it frustrating not to ejaculate? Well, it might be if you only had one non-ejaculatory orgasm. But by the time you've had several – it could be six, twelve, twenty – you'll look upon ejaculation as frustrating, for bringing such rapture to an end. It's the *cumulative* effect of male multiple orgasms that is so stunning, not the effect of a single one.

HOW IT FEELS TO A WOMAN

It's not only the man who benefits from this style of sex. Let's see what's in it for you, the woman. You can:

- enjoy as many orgasms as you want until you're totally satisfied
- enjoy taking your partner to successive peaks of excitement beyond anything in 'normal' sex

- *have a partner who constantly desires you*
- *have sex as often as you wish*
- *enter a mystical state in which the boundaries between you and your partner (and possibly the entire universe) seem to break down – which is the aim of Tantric sex.*

STRENGTHENING THE PC MUSCLE FOR MEN (AND WOMEN)

Strengthening the PC muscle, as Dr Kothari's subject did, is a very good idea, but not because of its potential to cut off the flow of semen. Far better is to use the PC muscle to make ejaculation less likely in the first place. For the way to do that, once the muscle is strong enough, see 'The locking method' on p. 168. Just as important, the stronger your PC, the more powerful your orgasms will be (and the longer you'll be able to enjoy them into old age). And that applies to women too. In Chapter 2 we did some basic exercises. Now we're going to move on to something more sophisticated.

Exercise 1 – *mula bandha*
This is a daily exercise for both sexes (and also a position, as described in Chapter 10).

- **Step 1:** *Sit comfortably and focus attention on the anus.*
- **Step 2:** *Inhale half a lungful of air and hold the breath.*
- **Step 3:** *Slowly contract the anal muscles until you have the feeling of retracting your anus up inside you. If you're a man you should feel this pulling your testicles and making your penis twitch, while if you're a woman your vaginal lips should twitch.*
- **Step 4:** *Release the contraction, take in a little air and then breathe out completely.*
- **Step 5:** *Repeat ten times, building up to 60 repetitions at the end of three months.*

Insight
If you're bothered by the word 'anus' try not to be. In Tantra, as I'm stressing throughout the book, every part of

the body is holy. And from a Western pragmatic perspective, you need to regard your body as a tool of your mind, to be trained, controlled and directed.

Exercise 2 – *vajroli mudra*
In its extreme form, *vajroli mudra* involves a man inserting a catheter (not recommended) but this simplified exercise applies to both men and women.

▶ **Step 1:** *Sit comfortably and focus attention on the urethral sphincter (the valve you would contract to hold back or cut off the flow of urine).*
▶ **Step 2:** *Inhale half a lungful of air and hold the breath.*
▶ **Step 3:** *Slowly contract the urethral sphincter. At first this may seem to be the same as* mula bandha *but the whole aim is to be able to manipulate the anal and urethral muscles separately. That will come with practice. If you're a man you should see your penis move. If you're a woman and insert a finger into your vagina you should feel the muscles contract around it.*
▶ **Step 4:** *Release the contraction, take in a little air and then breathe out completely.*
▶ **Step 5:** *Repeat ten times, building up to 60 repetitions at the end of three months.*

Initially, you may find that there's no difference between *mula bandha* and *vajroli mudra* because all your pelvic floor muscles operate together as a unit, especially when the contraction is very forceful. Spend a little time every day just lightly trying to contract the anus without the urethral sphincter, and vice versa. Quite soon you should find you can control the muscles separately and that's going to be important as you move on to more advanced sexual techniques.

Women have a particular advantage in PC muscle strengthening because they can easily introduce a resistance into their vaginas, such as the Kegel devices, first invented by Dr Arnold Kegel back in 1947 as a way of tackling urinary stress incontinence. Look for a model capable of providing different levels of resistance. But thousands of years ago women were inserting 'stone eggs' and using their muscles to move them up and down, not simply to strengthen the vagina but also to develop *control*. These kinds of exercises are known in India as *sahajoli* and I'll have more to say about them in Chapter 10. By the way, nowadays stainless steel is more popular than stone.

Learning to orgasm without ejaculation

To enjoy orgasm without ejaculation it would help if we knew exactly what it is that triggers the expulsion of semen. Unfortunately we don't. The debate is over whether ejaculation is triggered by the increased pressure of semen in the duct system or whether it's triggered by excitation in the brain/spinal cord reaching a certain threshold. We don't have complete proof but since 1990 we've had a pretty good idea. Three researchers (Gerstenberg, Levin and Wagner) conducted various trials and concluded it was 'unlikely' that the trigger came from 'distention by the semen of any internal organs'. Rather, it seems probable that the signal comes from the brain.

The desire to ejaculate during lovemaking is incredibly powerful. That's how evolution works. Men who had that drive reproduced the most successfully. To subvert nature, we need to condition the brain, and therefore the mind, to something different.

You can test the power of your mind in sex very easily. Self-stimulate until you're close to ejaculating. Then cease all physical stimulation and, instead, introduce mental stimulation. Visualize the sexiest scene you can imagine and, at the same time, say something out loud that really excites you. Undoubtedly you'll ejaculate…by the power of your mind.

WHAT YOU'RE AIMING FOR

Let me now try to explain what you're aiming for. To return to John Humphrey Noyes' analogy of the waterfall (see previous chapter), we're no longer going to paddle around in the calmer part of the river. We're going to row our boats right to the very edge of the falls, the point at which most men are swept over, and we're going to hang there as if suspended by a rope, enjoying the thrill as long as we want. Even more amazing, after revelling in the euphoria, we're going to paddle *back* against the current and safely return to the bank, ready to repeat the whole experience as soon as we like.

Have you ever noticed, when masturbating or making love, that there's a tiny moment, a mere fraction of a second before the PNR, that you simultaneously feel a delicious sensation in your genitals and a hit of happy chemicals in your brain, like a sort of mental orgasm? Most men, in fact, have never isolated that fragment. It all gets lost in the confusion of the ejaculatory orgasm. But if you ever have experienced that moment as something distinct, you'll understand at once. This is the very edge of the waterfall. Your goal is to, as it were, almost stop time at that pre-PNR moment – to lengthen the moment of extreme pleasure that precedes the PNR and to increase its intensity even more. Just as your body is on the very verge of ejaculating so, using the various techniques I'll be explaining, you prevent that ejaculation taking place. You *trick* your body. Your body is so convinced that the ejaculation is going to happen that it goes ahead and pumps those mind-altering chemicals into your brain anyway. For a few seconds you revel in that 'hit'. Then, as it starts to wane, you allow just the tiniest re-stimulation. Again chemicals are pumped into your brain and again you halt the ejaculation. And so it goes on, over and over again, pumping your brain, as it were, fuller and fuller of those bliss-inducing, mind-altering chemicals.

Now, orgasm without ejaculation obviously doesn't feel like a standard ejaculatory orgasm. In the first place, there's not that sense of relief. Rather than experiencing an intense craving that is resolved by the pumping out of semen, the desire continues unabated. At first that can seem like a negative but, in time, you'll be astounded that you could ever have felt that way, because now, instead, you'll desire your partner more in every way, desire sex with her more and be capable of more sex. It's also true that the orgasmic muscular contractions will be fewer and less powerful. Initially, that too will seem disappointing. But as your 'paddling' skill increases, you'll be able to experience the pre-PNR moment again and again, each time releasing more and more chemicals into your brain. It's the cumulative effect of these chemicals that, quite soon, overtakes the foregone pleasure of the single ejaculatory orgasm. And the longer you go on, the more you'll 'blow your mind'.

> ## Insight
> The first time I experienced Tantric sex including the withholding of ejaculation was one of the most beautiful, powerful and mystical events in my life. There was none of the fatigue, no reduction in my desire, none of the disappointment that something is over, no loss of energy and, instead, there was a joyful sense of connection not only with my partner but with the whole universe. And it lasted the whole of the next day.

MIND TRAINING

What you, as the man, have to do first of all is resolve that, no matter what happens, you will not ejaculate. No matter how excited you feel, no matter how excited your partner becomes, no matter how much she wants you to come, *you will not ejaculate*. Think of your semen, your sex drive and your sexual energy as incredibly precious things that, under no circumstances, can be frittered away. Think of 'proper' sex as sex without ejaculation. Think of ejaculation as failure.

Of course, there will be occasions on which you make a decision *to* ejaculate. But this is a decision that must always be taken in advance. It's no good saying you'll see how you feel when the moment comes. That just won't work. You must be clear in your mind as to when you're having a non-ejaculatory session, and when you're having an ejaculatory session – and your partner must be clear, as well.

Reprogramming your mind
I've already made the point that ejaculation control is more an issue of mind than matter. So that's where we'll start. Something that's quite effective is to *visualize* yourself making love without

ejaculating. Make your visualization as detailed as possible. Really see, hear, feel, touch and taste everything. Experience your partner having orgasm after orgasm while you remain in perfect control.

Visualizations like this are easy to fit into even the busiest day, so this is something you can repeat often to build up the effect. But the way to maximize the power of your mind is to employ self-hypnosis.

Many of the early Tantric practitioners would have been no strangers to trance, but nothing like this technique seems to have been used by them for ejaculation control. This particular method of self-hypnosis is attributed to the American hypnotherapist Betty Erickson, the wife of Milton Erickson, founding president of the American Society for Clinical Hypnosis. (The same approach can also be used for all kinds of other things.)

Have a go

▶ **Step 1:** *Get yourself comfortable in a place you won't be disturbed. It's not a good idea to lie on the bed because you might fall asleep. But you could sit up on the bed supported by pillows, or arrange yourself in a nice, comfy chair.*

▶ **Step 2:** *Decide the length of time you wish to spend in self-hypnosis. Initially I'd suggest trying 10 minutes. That should give you enough time to achieve a deep state of trance without feeling anxiety about 'wasting' time. So, having got comfortable, you should say something like this: 'I am now going to hypnotize myself for 10 minutes.' You might like to append the actual time by adding '...which means I will come out of self-hypnosis at 7.30 p.m.(or whatever).'*

▶ **Step 3:** *This is a key step because it's where you state the purpose of your hypnosis. The exact words aren't important. Something along these lines will do fine: 'I am entering into a trance for the purpose of allowing my unconscious mind to make the adjustments that will help me stay in full control during sex so that I will not ejaculate.' Whatever you say, make sure it includes the message that you are inviting your unconscious to deal with the matter. You might also like to add some words of encouragement: '...will not ejaculate, even though I shall be as rigid as a bar of iron.'*

▶ **Step 4:** *State how you want to feel when you come out of your trance. It may be you will simply want to experience your 'normal waking state'. Or it might be you will immediately want to make use of the change your unconscious has made. In that case you might say, for example, '...and as I come out of my trance I will feel full of desire for my partner and confident in my ability to give her multiple orgasms.'*

▶ **Step 5:** *This is the actual process of self-hypnosis. Basically you're going to engage your three main representational systems in turn to bring the trance about. In the first part of the process you will be noting things you can actually see, hear and feel* in the room where you are. *In the second part you will be noting things you can see, hear and feel* in an imaginary scene.

Below is a diagram that represents the whole process. In the diagram, V = Visual system, A = Auditory system, and K = Kinaesthetic system.

```
V                   V                   V
A                   A                   A
K                   K                   K
         V                   V
         A                   A
         K                   K
                   V
                   A
                   K
         (External reality)
---------------------------------------------
         (Internal visualization)
                   V
                   A
                   K
         V                   V
         A                   A
         K                   K
V                   V                   V
A                   A                   A
K                   K                   K
```

In this process, some people talk to themselves internally, but I recommend that *you say everything out loud*. For that reason, you'll want to be in a private place. You might imagine that you'd 'wake' yourself up but, in fact, the sound of your own voice, done the right way, will intensify the effect. (If, however, speaking out loud doesn't work for you then by all means speak internally.)

Have a go

▶ **Step 1:** *From your comfortable position, look at some small thing in the room in front of you and say out loud what you are looking at. Choose things you can see without moving your head. For example, 'I am looking at the door handle.' Then, without rushing, focus on another small item. For example, 'I am now looking at a glass of water on the table.' Then move on to a third item. For example, 'I am looking at the light switch.' When you have your three visual references, move on.*

▶ **Step 2:** *Switch attention to sounds and, in the same way, note one after another until you have three, each time saying out loud what you're hearing. Then move on to the next step.*

▶ **Step 3:** *Note things that you can feel with your body. For example, you might say, 'I can feel the seat pressing against my buttocks.' When you have your three, move on.*

▶ **Step 4:** *Now repeat steps 1 to 3 but with only two items for each sense, that's to say, two images, two sounds and two feelings. They must be different from the ones you used before. This time speak a little more slowly.*

▶ **Step 5:** *Again repeat steps 1 to 3, but with only one item per sense, that's to say, one image, one sound and one feeling. Again, they must be different from any that have gone before. Speak even more slowly.*

▶ **Step 6:** *Close your eyes, if they're not already closed, and visualize making Tantric-style love to your partner.*

▶ **Step 7:** *Using this imagined scene, go through the same process you already used for the real scene, but beginning with just one example of each of the three senses, that is, one image, one sound and one feeling. For example, you might say: 'I see my* lingam *in my partner's yoni...I hear my partner cry out as she comes...I feel my* lingam *rigid and yet under complete control...' When you've done that, increase to two examples* *of each sense and then three. (Three is usually enough, but if you've stipulated a lengthy session you may need to continue with your fantasy scene by going on to name four images, sounds and feelings, or five or even more.) Remember, each example must be different. You'll probably find you're automatically speaking very slowly now but, if not, make a point of slowing your voice down more and more.*

▶ **Step 8:** *After the allotted time you should begin to come out of trance automatically. But it may help to announce, 'I'll count to three and when I reach three I'll be (whatever you said in Step 4).' Don't worry about getting 'stuck' in a trance. That won't happen. You may feel a little woozy for a while. If so, don't drive a car or do anything demanding until you're sure you're okay to do so.*

Your unconscious will not only deal with the stated purpose of your self-hypnosis all the time you're in trance but, probably, afterwards, too. Even so you may need to repeat the procedure a few times to obtain an enduring result.

Reprogramming your body

Every man is used to 'stop-go' – that's to say, easing back when excitement builds too fast and getting going again once the danger of ejaculation has passed. But most men never get anywhere near the optimum level of excitement before they 'stop'. They, as it were, paddle their boats to the start of the rapids then dash back to the safety of calm water. At some point they can't resist the current any longer – they don't want to – and over the falls they go.

So how do we physically keep our boats hanging on the edge of the falls? Having developed the necessary mental resolve through the mind exercises above, we:

▶ *refine our 'stop-go' skills to the optimum*
▶ *introduce breath control*
▶ *employ the 'locking method'*
▶ *redirect sexual energy*
▶ *use the 'superpanting' technique.*

So let's start the physical training. You'll probably want to do this on your own but, if you feel like company there's no reason you can't sometimes practise together with your partner when she also feels like masturbating.

Practice makes perfect

Here's one of the keys to the whole thing. Learning control is not like learning to ride a bicycle. It's not a question of acquiring a knack that you'll have for all time. It's far more like any form of physical conditioning. You have to train regularly otherwise your level of skill diminishes. Therefore, aim to masturbate without ejaculating at least once a day and aim for a session of 30 minutes to one hour every week.

Refining stop-go

Begin self-stimulating in your usual way. Remind yourself that you will not ejaculate, no matter how tempting it seems. When you get close to the PNR (but not too close) cease all stimulation. That means you must stop physical stimulation, stop looking at your partner's body (if you are), stop looking at pornography (if you are), stop fantasizing (if you are), and stop tensing the muscles of your body (if you are). Don't do anything at all that could possibly generate any sexual feelings. Let the excitement die away a little and then, when you feel it's safe, resume stimulation. Keep on like this but don't get right up against the PNR until about 20 or 30 minutes have gone by. By that time your genitals will probably feel fatigued and you should find it easier to keep control. If you do go over the edge, don't worry. Just enjoy it and try again another time.

Breath control

Once you've worked up a head of steam in stop-go you can start adding the special techniques. For this one, while you're self-stimulating, breathe very consciously, steadily, deeply and calmly, allowing rather more time for breathing out than breathing in. You should immediately notice that you feel more controlled.

The locking method

Kneel on the bed and self-stimulate some more. As you approach the PNR, arch your back, contract your PC muscle (which you should be strengthening from previous exercises) and pull your abdominal muscles in towards your spine as tightly as you can. You should find that, for as long as you can keep all those particular muscles tensed, you can carry on moderate self-stimulation (or thrusting) without breaching the PNR. It seems that, along with various other organs, your prostate is compressed and prevented from pulsating.

This is the same technique as employed by Dr Kothari's subject (see p. 156) but *before* ejaculation, not after. Why not do it after? Because it then only reduces the volume of semen and shortens but doesn't eradicate the refractory period (the period you have to wait before you can have sex again). So it's more effective to do this before ejaculation. The most extreme version of physically obstructing the flow of semen, known as the **'million dollar point'** technique, is not something I recommend but I describe it in the factbox below so you'll have a more complete knowledge of the various techniques.

The million dollar point and the squeeze technique

This method has been called the 'million dollar point' because wealthy men were said to be willing to pay Indian gurus that much for the 'secret'. I'll tell you it for much less but I wouldn't recommend it. The idea is to press hard on the perineum with two or three fingers up towards the prostate gland immediately as the PNR has been breached. The point at which the pressure needs to be applied is the indentation that lies between the testicles and the anus. If you search around there you'll find it quite easily. But there are various problems with this method:

▶ *It can hurt.*
▶ *It risks damaging the urethra and other parts of the sexual apparatus.*

- *It only reduces the refractory period, but does not eliminate it.*
- *The semen has to go somewhere, which may be backwards into the bladder (what's known as 'retrograde ejaculation'), possibly causing some damage to the proximal sphincter.*
- *The pleasure of orgasm and ejaculation will be reduced and there may be no pleasure at all.*
- *For a reduced refractory period, it just isn't worth it, in my view, especially since there are alternatives.*

The million dollar point shouldn't be confused with the squeeze technique which was developed by the sex researchers Masters and Johnson for the treatment of premature ejaculation. Ever since then it's been quoted by various sexologists as a means of halting ejaculation once it's started. However, that's a complete misconception. Masters and Johnson themselves wrote that their method 'should not be used, however, at the moment of ejaculatory inevitability'. There are two genuine versions. In the 'easy' version, the man withdraws from the vagina from time to time and his partner then puts the pad of her thumb on his frenulum, with her first and second fingers on the opposite side, and squeezes. In the 'advanced' version, either the woman or the man squeezes the base of the penis for about four seconds, with the thumb on the urethra (that is, squeezes from front to back, not side to side). From the point of view of a man who doesn't suffer premature ejaculation, this is quite valueless since *anything* that interrupts stimulation is bound to cause the PNR to recede.

Redirecting sexual energy
If you've forgotten about *Kundalini* or 'sexual energy', refer back to Chapter 2. The idea of this technique is to divert *Kundalini* into some part or parts of the body where it won't trigger ejaculation.

Imagine that you've generated enormous energy in your genitals and you've directed some of that energy up into your brain and, therefore, your mind, so as to achieve the highly altered state of consciousness that is the aim of Tantric sex. As you continue to generate energy, so you now have to divert it somewhere else, otherwise ejaculation will be triggered. Exactly *where* is something you'll have to experiment with, because everybody is different. A traditional Tantric technique was to screw up the eyes and grind the teeth, but that's not a lot of fun. Biting your partner's tongue (gently), or pressing your tongue against hers, works for some people and can be very sexy. Others report that tongues are *too* sexy and can themselves be triggers. The anus can also be a Janus (the Roman god depicted with two faces looking in opposite directions). Stimulation of the anus close to the PNR is so exciting that it's certain to send you over the falls. On the other hand, if you begin directing energy there well before the PNR, then it has the capacity to draw a great deal of attention from the genitals. Safer places to direct energy are the nipples (which can benefit from being sensitized in this way), the neck, the ears and the toes.

'Superpanting' – the ultimate technique

I'm now going to teach you the ultimate Tantric technique for unlimited, orgasmic, non-ejaculatory sex. It doesn't require you to do anything at all complicated. In fact, it sounds so simple that, at first, you probably won't even believe me. But when you try it you'll see for yourself.

▶ **Step 1:** *As soon as you feel you're about to ejaculate, stick your tongue out and down and, with your mouth open, pant with forceful exhalations of one or two seconds each.*

▶ **Step 2:** *Get rid of that air from your lungs as if it's toxic. This isn't panting like a contented dog – it's 'superpanting'. Really be dramatic about it. And keep on until the urge has passed. Ok, you may not look at your most attractive, but when you come to do this during sex with your partner, she may be pulling a few faces of her own.*

▶ **Step 3:** *Now how do you feel? It's magic, isn't it! Just a moment ago you were about to ejaculate and, suddenly, you're back* *in the calmer waters. How does it work? There seem to be several possible mechanisms not fully unravelled by science, but there's one you can clearly see for yourself if you go over to the mirror. Stimulate yourself until you see your scrotum tighten up against your groin and then repeat the superpanting. You'll see your testicles redescend – just as if, in fact, your partner had pulled them away from your body, as some sexologists recommend (see the Insight below). But there's no need for any physical pulling of the testicles because it can all be done under the control of the cremaster muscle. When you're very excited (or when you clench your PC muscle) the cremaster contracts and pulls the scrotum up. When you superpant in the way described (or consciously relax your PC muscle), the cremaster extends and the scrotum drops.*

Once you've mastered the techniques such that you can masturbate for half an hour or more, close to the PNR but without ejaculating, then you're ready to try the techniques with your partner.

Insight

It's a fact that, as ejaculation approaches, the cremaster muscle hauls the scrotum tight up against the groin. Some sexologists therefore recommend that you should get your partner to pull your testicles down to halt ejaculation. In my experience the effect is often quite the reverse. Feeling your partner's hand on your testicles at the critical moment is all that's needed to guarantee that ejaculation *will* take place. When she hears you superpant, you want your partner to do nothing at all.

Multiple orgasms with your partner

Hopefully you've now mastered all the various techniques while masturbating, and you're about to have Tantric sex with your partner. You've made up your mind that, for this session, you're going to enjoy multiple orgasms and you won't ejaculate at the end.

But there's a new problem. You may have got pretty good control of yourself but you're now about to make love to another person and you don't have control of *her*. So: *you have to tell your partner what you're planning and she needs to be in full agreement and very happy to co-operate.*

POSITION

Quite a few sexperts recommend beginning with one of the more static woman-on-top poses (as used in the previous chapter) but I strongly disagree. If it's difficult for you to gauge the amount of stimulation that will keep you right on the PNR without going over, then it's almost impossible for your partner. How is she to know exactly when to halt movement? What's more, woman-on-top positions can cause older men to lose some erection (due to gravity) resulting in more desperate, less controlled thrusting. It's far better to choose a position in which:

▶ *you can precisely judge the amount of stimulation and instantly increase or decrease it*
▶ *you can clearly communicate with your partner*
▶ *you can maintain a powerful erection.*

The best positions for multi-orgasmic beginners are therefore *samapada-uttana-bandha* and *vyomapada-uttana bandha*, squatting or kneeling between your partner's thighs (see Chapter 10).

Have a go
▶ **Step 1:** *Resolve that you will not ejaculate (and, if necessary, increase your willpower through visualization and self-hypnosis, as explained above).*
▶ **Step 2:** *Agree a sign that you will give for your partner to cease all movement and stimulation instantly. (The tiniest things can cause a breach of the PNR, ranging from a contraction of the yoni to a 'taboo' word.) Probably the easiest signal is when she sees or hears you superpanting.*
▶ **Step 3:** *Prepare the room and yourselves in the usual Tantric way.*
▶ **Step 4:** *Arouse one another using the techniques of* nyasa *and* auparishtaka *as described in Chapters 5 and 6.*

- ▶ **Step 5:** *Unite* lingam *and* yoni *in the chosen position.*
- ▶ **Step 6:** *Excite one another, moving as you both wish, until the PNR is close.*
- ▶ **Step 7:** *You, the man, are now going to take full control of movement, using stop-go, breath control, the locking method, redirection of sexual energy and the superpanting technique to keep close to the PNR, without going over.*
- ▶ **Step 8:** *Revel in each 'hit' of 'happy' chemicals, driving* Kundalini *higher and higher and transforming the energy, through the chakras (see Chapter 2) to achieve oneness with your partner and, if that's how you want to feel, oneness with the universe.*
- ▶ **Step 9:** *Continue as long as you both wish (see p. 174) but at least try to continue intercourse for half an hour and don't stop, if you can help it, until you reach a state of* ananda.
- ▶ **Step 10:** *After withdrawing the* lingam *from the* yoni, *remain together cuddling and basking in the afterglow for at least 15 minutes.*

Your initial attempts at multi-orgasmic sex with your partner may necessarily be a little 'selfish'. That is, you'll be concentrating a lot on not ejaculating rather than on your partner. She may get a bit frustrated if the build-up to her own orgasms is halted by you. Make up for that by playing with her clitoris to orgasm, or encouraging her to do so (when it's 'safe'). Later, when you have a higher level of skill, you should be able to give your partner numerous orgasms directly as a result of your thrusting.

THE LUBRICANT TRICK

There's one additional technique you might like to experiment with when you're practising multiple orgasms with your partner, and that's lubricants. Normally they're used to *increase* sexual pleasure, especially when natural lubrication isn't adequate. But they can also be used to *decrease* stimulation. Excessive lubricant, for example, can reduce friction and, therefore, the urge to ejaculate. Silicone lubricants are so slippery that they're particularly useful in this way. And very thick lubricants like KY jelly, lavishly applied, can act as a sort of barrier between *lingam* and *yoni*. Lubricants are a very personal thing so buy half a dozen different kinds and test the effects they're capable of producing. (Remember that only silicone and water-based lubricants should be used with latex condoms.)

_____

How long to continue

In 'normal' sex, the average couple stops when the man ejaculates. Unless he's young or unusually virile, he won't have either the inclination or ability to continue – so there's a clear end. But if the man doesn't ejaculate, when do you stop? It may sound like a silly question, but the problem is that it's difficult to be the one who says, 'That's enough.'

At one time, men were criticized for being unable to satisfy their partners. The average man ejaculated so quickly, his lover didn't even have a single orgasm. It's tempting, therefore, for modern men to assume that their lovers will be delighted to continue sex for hours on end. In fact, the orgasmic capacity of *some* women is awesome. The record seems to be 134 orgasms in an hour. But that is far from the sort of lovemaking that most women want.

In my focus groups, I haven't yet encountered a woman who was thrilled by the idea of Tantric intercourse continuing for even an hour, let alone several hours. For a start, it's a mistake to imagine that the inside of a woman's vagina is similar to the outside of a man's penis. It's actually far more delicate and less able to withstand lengthy friction, so women tend to feel sore long before men do. But there's another problem. Although the science is still a little vague, it seems any kind of genital stimulation causes women to produce prolactin. And prolactin (as we saw in the previous chapter) kills sexual desire. Men, by contrast, seem to produce prolactin mainly when they ejaculate, so by having sex without ejaculation they escape it. So we've gone from one imbalance (women wanting longer intercourse than men were capable of) to the opposite (men wanting longer intercourse than women are capable of).

Lubricant can help with mechanical chafing, but the only way to stop a woman producing prolactin is to stop stimulating her genitals. If you, the man, discover that you become capable of far longer sessions than your partner, the solution, then, is for your partner to stimulate you orally, with her fingers, between her breasts, and between her thighs *before* moving on to intercourse.

So, if you, the man, are intent on continuing intercourse for a long time, you're probably putting a lot of pressure on your partner. She's going to have to be the 'killjoy' every time by saying she's had enough, and that's not good for your Tantric sex life together. So be observant and when you detect that your partner's excitement is waning (you'll note less energy in her *yoni*, for example) then *you* be the one to suggest bringing the session to an end.

FREQUENCY OF MULTI-ORGASMIC SEX

The frequency with which you, the man, have sex will have a direct bearing on your ability to control ejaculation. If you have multi-orgasmic sex at regular, frequent intervals with a partner with whom you have a high degree of complicity, then you'll find it relatively easy to keep control. By contrast, if you don't have a regular partner and, consequently, have sex at infrequent, irregular intervals, the compulsion to ejaculate very quickly is bound to be enormous. In that case, it will help if, in addition to your non-ejaculatory 'training sessions', you also allow yourself to ejaculate from time to time when masturbating. How often depends on your sexual make-up – that's something for you to discover. But it would be a mistake to assume that lots of masturbatory ejaculation will make you a better lover by making it harder to ejaculate with your partner. On the contrary, if too much ejaculation means you have to thrust more quickly and more vigorously to maintain erection, then you won't be in control. Paradoxically, you'll have maximum control when your erection is dependably rigid.

THE BALANCE BETWEEN EJACULATORY AND NON-EJACULATORY SESSIONS

Once you, the man, have learned to be multi-orgasmic you'll always want to be multi-orgasmic. Why would you not be?

But you won't always want to ejaculate. So it's quite likely your partner will want to experience simultaneous orgasm/ejaculation more often than you. You'll need to work out a new sexual rhythm between you. Here are a few things to bear in mind:

▶ *If you don't ejaculate, you'll be capable of having sex every day, or even more often.*
▶ *If you have daily non-ejaculatory 'quickies', you'll probably find the sexual tension building with each session so that it's harder and harder to keep control. You may begin to feel frustrated, which is the opposite of what's intended.*
▶ *In order not to feel frustrated, it's important to have regular, lengthy Tantric sessions. Even without ejaculation, there's always some sexual fluid that seeps out, thus reducing tension. What's more, long sessions fatigue the whole sexual apparatus leading to a quiet, mystical tranquility.*

THE WOMAN'S VIEW

So your partner is in training to master multiple orgasms. That's going to change his experience of sex, but it's also going to change yours. Quite a lot. We've already looked at some of the issues that concern you as a couple. Now let's look at some of the issues that particularly affect you as a woman.

First of all, while he's gaining in experience, he's not going to be concentrating on you as he should. That will improve. He's also going to make some 'mistakes'. That's to say, he's going to ejaculate when he didn't intend to. Because he won't have been expecting it, you won't have been expecting it either. That may mess up your plans for a final simultaneous orgasm. Well, these things happen. Enjoy what you can and keep in mind that once he's mastered the skills you're going to have a wonderful multi-orgasmic time yourself.

Something that may bother you is the thought that if he's not ejaculating he's not really getting excited. You may think he's being too controlled. You may wonder why you're not turning him on. All those kind of ideas are simply the result of conditioning. Stop thinking of your partner's ejaculation as normal and, instead, see it as occasional. Say to yourself that:

- *ejaculation is for reproduction*
- *non-ejaculation is for sexual pleasure.*

I can assure you, your partner will be having the best time of his life and reaching a level of excitement far beyond anything he ever used to experience.

You may also feel like a killjoy when your vagina is telling you it's had enough and you now have to tell him. Well, in fact, don't worry about it at all. He'll already have had far more pleasure from his Tantric session than he ever would have got from a 'normal' session ending with ejaculation. And he'll know it.

> **Warning:** Non-ejaculation is not a substitute for your normal birth control methods. A little fluid will always seep out and may contain viable sperm.

Multiple orgasms for women

Shaktis are rather different to Shivas when it comes to multiple orgasms. They can enjoy them quite naturally without having to master special techniques. So why, you might be asking, aren't *I* having multiple orgasms? If you are asking that question, read on.

Years ago, women didn't have orgasms because they didn't expect to have orgasms (nor did their partners expect them to). Now things have progressed. The majority of women (about 90 per cent, according to some researchers) expect to orgasm and do. But only about a quarter expect to experience multiple orgasms and do. So the first thing to do is start expecting them. In fact, you almost certainly are multi-orgasmic and you just don't know it. The way to unlock your multi-orgasmic capacity is not through intercourse but through masturbation. Multi-orgasmic sex with a partner can wait until you're reliably multi-orgasmic on your own.

In my focus groups, some women talk of having to 'work' at their orgasms. They sometimes describe their efforts as 'desperate' and 'grubby'. One woman said she had managed a second orgasm but it had taken 'too long'. When I asked how long, she said '15 minutes'. These women all have an attitude problem. If you think spending 15 minutes on sex is 'too long' then you're never going to enjoy yourself.

Take note, too, of the word 'grubby'. If you're going to become multi-orgasmic, you have to get rid of any negative attitudes like this and, instead, get more Tantric. In Tantric sex, almost nothing pleasurable is taboo. Breaking taboos is all part of expanding consciousness. Don't be embarrassed about self-stimulation. When masturbating you should be:

- *joyful*
- *uninhibited*
- *expansive*
- *inventive*
- *relaxed*.

How much you enjoy sex with your partner doesn't depend solely on your partner. He can't magically make your body do things it doesn't know how to do. If you want to experience the outer reaches of ecstasy your body has to be trained – and you're the best person to do it. Masturbation isn't an option. It's essential. And, in fact, you can also discover a surprising amount about your partner's body by exploring your own because men's and women's bodies are far more alike than different.

Have a go
Have your one orgasm by your usual method of masturbation, but don't have it in the back of your mind that you'll settle for one. Be optimistic. Now simply continue to play with your clitoris.

It may be that you'll surprise yourself by having a second orgasm without doing anything else. And a third.

If not, you're going to have to do something unusual, something extra, to get those additional orgasms. Later on, special techniques may not be necessary. In fact, women who are multi-orgasmic say that, after the first, orgasms come more easily. For now, while you're training your body to produce multiple orgasms, you may have to throw everything at it, up to but not quite including the kitchen sink. The first thing is the power of your mind and the advice is the same as for men. That is, visualize yourself having orgasm after orgasm and, if that's not enough, use the Betty Erickson self-hypnosis method (see pp. 163–5).

After that, you have to raise the erotic temperature higher than you ever have before and continue longer than you ever have before. Don't forget, either, that orgasm is a release of tension. Before you can release that tension you first of all have to build it. Here are a few ideas:

- ▶ *Put on some sensual, very rhythmic music.*
- ▶ *Strip completely naked, if you're not already.*
- ▶ *Relax. Give yourself an hour to succeed.*
- ▶ *Rub yourself all over with some body oil.*
- ▶ *Use a vibrator.*
- ▶ *Try different positions.*
- ▶ *Stimulate other places in addition to your clitoris – the entrance to your vagina, your G-spot area, your anus, your nipples – whatever excites you.*
- ▶ *Focus attention on whatever part of your body you're playing with.*
- ▶ *Increase the blood flow by spanking yourself.*
- ▶ *Fantasize.*
- ▶ *Speak your fantasy out loud.*
- ▶ *Try masturbating while watching an erotic video or DVD.*
- ▶ *Try masturbating in front of a mirror or while making a video of yourself or watching yourself on a TV monitor.*
- ▶ *Make plenty of noise.*

PROBLEMS

The sex researcher Shere Hite found quite a lot of women who said they could only orgasm with their legs together. I suspect the women who said they couldn't orgasm with their legs apart simply didn't have their legs *far enough* apart. A comfortable distance just doesn't generate sufficient tension for women who don't orgasm easily. On your back, practise increasing and decreasing physical tension in your legs by opening and closing them and holding them up in the air. See what effect that has on your excitement. It should increase and decrease in step. Or bring your knees back as close as you can to your ears. Or try kneeling with your thighs open and lean back as far as you can – use some pillows to support you. The more physical tension you create (without actual discomfort), the better.

Some women report that they'd like to carry on stimulating themselves and believe they would have further orgasms but their clitorises become too sensitive to touch after the first orgasm. If this happens to you, try continuing the stimulation above your clitoris or to the side or try some of your other erogenous places. Above all, continue the stimulation in your mind.

If, after all that, you still didn't have multiple orgasms, don't give up. Time is on your side. The more sex you have, the more likely you are to become multi-orgasmic. The body learns and responds by, for example, increasing the density of blood vessels in the genitals. Sexually active women naturally become more orgasmic as they get older. Interestingly, some women experience their first multiple orgasms whilst pregnant. Every week, set aside one hour for 'multiple orgasm training' and keep on until you succeed.

Multiple orgasms with your partner

If you have a non-Tantric partner (hopefully not the case) who only wants to orgasm/ejaculate once himself, as is usual, it may be that he assumes you only need to orgasm once as well. Quite probably, because of him, you've accepted the idea that one is enough for you too.

Once you've mastered multi-orgasms on your own, you need to let your partner know that you want to try for more with him. Don't be embarrassed about it. Some women are afraid they'll be thought of as nymphomaniacs, but most men respond very positively to the idea of 'giving' their partners multiple orgasms. The more orgasms a woman has, the more macho the man feels. The more you enjoy yourself, the more he's going to enjoy himself.

If you do have a Tantric partner (hopefully the case) then, of course, he will want you to have plenty of orgasms. Shiva knows it's going to be difficult for you to enjoy lengthy Tantric sex sessions if you don't have lots. Apart from which, it's with each orgasm that you, like Shiva, will be pushing *Kundalini* higher and higher, transforming the energy into oneness with your partner and, if you wish, oneness with the universe (see Chapter 2).

How many could you have? Well, I've already mentioned the record of 134 in an hour. And a few rare women have multiple orgasms that seem to be one continuous orgasm (only scientific instruments can make the distinction) lasting for perhaps a minute, an experience known as 'status orgasmus'. But these are extremes and the majority of multi-orgasmic women say three to six is about right.

Have a go
  ▶ Step 1: *When having Tantric sex with your partner, make full use of the knowledge you gained about your body during your masturbation sessions. Don't forget to visualize those chakras (traditional or personal, as you prefer) to transform the sexual energy with each orgasm.*
  ▶ Step 2: *After nyasa (see Chapter 5), give yourself one orgasm with a vibrator or fingers while your partner watches – most men enjoy that.*
  ▶ Step 3: *Have a second orgasm from your partner giving you oral sex.*

▶ **Step 4:** *Have a third orgasm with* lingam *and* yoni *united, perhaps in a goddess-on-top position (see Chapter 10) so you have complete control. You can also play with yourself at the same time.*

▶ **Step 5:** *Go for a fourth orgasm in a rear-entry position.*

▶ **Step 6:** *Let your partner have a rest while you self-stimulate to a fifth orgasm.*

▶ **Step 7:** *Unite* lingam *and* yoni *once more, perhaps this time in a Shiva-on-top position. Remember that you can increase tension by opening your legs as widely as possible and holding them up off the bed. During intercourse this is also highly stimulating, visually, for your partner. Or get your knees back by your ears, again extremely erotic. By now you should be in such an altered state that your body and your partner's seem to be one. Now have your sixth orgasm and experience* ananda.

The little scenario above is just to give an idea. It's not something you have to follow exactly. The main difference between multiple orgasms in 'normal' sex and multiple orgasms in Tantric sex, is the way the sexual energy is progressively converted into an experience of *ananda*.

THE MAN'S VIEW

There are several special things you can do to help your partner enjoy multiple orgasms with you. The most important is to encourage her to play with herself however she wants during intercourse. Don't go believing that a 'real man' can 'give' a woman as many orgasms as she wants. Her orgasms are not *your* sole responsibility. They're hers, too. If she wants to, say, fondle her nipples or rub her clitoris during intercourse then that's fine. Skilful lovers understand that. Encourage her.

Be willing to try a variety of positions and techniques. It's true that some parts of the body can take a long time to develop a response (there are woman who orgasm after an hour of nipple stimulation) but, as a general rule, if something isn't working, switch to something else.

Remember that nothing is more exciting than knowing you're exciting your partner. So show your excitement. It's infectious.

And don't forget to ask her what she wants you to do. Hopefully she'll tell you what worked when she was masturbating. But if she's reluctant to respond to such a direct request then you'll just have to be very sensitive to her reactions.

Simultaneous orgasms

If you're both going to ejaculate/orgasm as the climax to your lovemaking then it would be the aim of all Tantrikas (and, indeed, most couples) to do so simultaneously. Some lovers find this extremely easy, while others find it frustratingly elusive.

In Tantric sex, simultaneous orgasm (for simplicity let's call it that rather than simultaneous ejaculation/orgasm) has always been important since it was believed to cause the 'sexual fluids' to mix together to create a powerful, magical potion (see Chapter 6). It was equally believed that the energy of the combined orgasms could be used in magic, a belief that persists in so-called 'witchcraft' to this day (see the factbox on p. 186).

If you've read this chapter so far and mastered the various exercises, you shouldn't have too much trouble reaching simultaneous orgasm. The training for men is to learn to withhold ejaculation, while the training for women is more or less the opposite, that is, being able to have orgasm after orgasm, more or less at will. If her partner 'misses' one orgasm he can always 'catch' the next one. That was all explained above, but there are a few extra 'tricks' that can help.

COMMUNICATION

The first 'trick' is communication. It's amazing how many couples have sex in near silence, and that's no good. Don't be afraid that talking about sex will somehow spoil it. The reverse is the case. The first thing you need to communicate about is the kind of session you envisage. If one of you is thinking of a 'quickie' (not actually Tantric) and the other of a 'slowie' then it would hardly be surprising if you didn't come together. If you permanently have very different ideas, you obviously need to get down to some serious discussion.

All the time you're having sex, maintain the communication. Obviously your senses will tell you a great deal, but it's still a good idea to ask a few questions. 'Are you getting close to orgasm?' 'Do you want to come soon?' You must make it clear when you'd like more stimulation, when you'd like less stimulation, when you'd like different stimulation, and, above all, when you feel you're approaching orgasm/ejaculation. Make it plain in good time. Don't announce it and then come one second later. Your partner won't have time to respond. When you feel the sensations building up, tell your partner so he or she can tune in to that and become excited by your excitement. And don't only rely on words. At this stage, sounds can be even better.

TRICKS WITH FANTASIES

The mind, as we've seen, is hugely important in sex. Above, we looked at ways of using the mind to control ejaculation. Here we're going to do more or less the opposite. We're going to use it to unleash a storm of excitement and bring on orgasm/ejaculation for the partner who is 'lagging behind'.

Ask your partner to recount his or her fantasies and then join in those fantasies, feeding them back. You need to be fairly uninhibited for this and that's all part of Tantric sex. But don't think you necessarily have to use Tantric fantasies. The original Tantrikas revelled in all kinds of practices that were taboo in their culture and you can do the same for your culture. For example:

> He: *Tell me what really turns you on.*
> She: *I get excited by the idea of people watching.*
> He (taking up the theme): *Yes, we could have sex on the beach tomorrow.*

She: At first they'd hardly notice...
He: But then as I stripped off your bikini they'd realize...
She: And they'd get round us in a circle...
He: And they'd all be thinking how sexy you look...

You can also use 'fantasies' to move energy around (see *Redirecting sexual energy* above). A common mistake that men make when they think they've lost control is to focus on their genitals. The effect is to send extra energy there, thus causing the ejaculation they hoped to escape. The correct response is to focus on somewhere else. By contrast, if you want to increase sexual excitement, you should focus on your genitals. For example, if you're a woman, it may help to create a mental image of your partner's penis thrusting in and out of your vagina while vaginal lubrication trickles down your thighs and your clitoris hardens with desire.

Finally, a highly effective trick for bringing someone very quickly back to Earth is to announce something like: 'I'm going to have to answer the telephone.' Obviously, it's a trick you can only get away with now and then.

A PHYSICAL TRICK FOR MEN

The easiest way for a man to calm down might appear to be to withdraw, but pulling back through the tightness of the vaginal lips can add that little extra stimulation that tips a man over. Given that the excited *yoni* actually balloons open in front of the cervix it's usually safer for the man to thrust *in* rather than pull *out*. Once excitement has died down a little it will then be safe to withdraw.

You, the man, can then watch while your partner plays with herself. Remember that no matter how good you are as a lover, you can never act with the precision that the owner of the body can. Alternatively, you can stimulate her with lips, fingers or a sex toy until she's close to orgasm. Once she's much more excited and you're a little less excited, unite *lingam* and *yoni* once more.

A PHYSICAL TRICK FOR MEN AND WOMEN

Wouldn't it be good if, in addition to all the other bits and pieces, there was a sort of 'orgasm/ejaculation button' you could press. Well, for a lot of men and women there is. It's called the anus. It's so packed with nerve endings, it's second only to the penis/clitoris. Yet it's neglected by many couples. In the next chapter we'll be putting that right.

Sex magick

Aleister Crowley (1875–1947), known in the popular press as 'the wickedest man in the world' and to himself as the 'Great Beast 666', was probably the most famous believer in the 'magical' power of orgasm. Although he never acknowledged his debt, it's very clear that his beliefs came from Tantric sex via his membership of organizations such as the Hermetic Order of the Golden Dawn (founded by William Westcott and MacGregor Mathers in 1887) and the German Ordo Templi Orientis (OTO), which translates as the 'Order of Eastern Templars' founded around 1895 by a wealthy German industrialist called Karl Kellner. The Golden Dawn was sufficiently benign to attract such members as the poet W. B. Yeats, but the OTO demanded rather more of its followers in sexual terms. Crowley, like the others, would invoke a god into himself during masturbation or intercourse and then, at orgasm, attempt to transfer his own consciousness into the god. Another technique was to concentrate on a talisman during sex and then anoint it with the 'elixir', which was the combination of 'the blood of the red lion' (semen) and the 'menstruum of the gluten' (the woman's sexual fluids).

But Crowley was the sort of man who preferred to lead his own magick order (the 'k' differentiates it from conjuring-type magic) and in the 1920s founded the Abbey of Thelema in Sicily to experiment in drug-fuelled sex. As he explained in his *Confessions*, he knew a 'secret, which is a scientific secret' which meant 'there would be nothing which the human imagination can conceive that could not be realized in practice'. That 'secret' was the power of sexual fluids and orgasm.

The fascinating thing is that, although the 'magicians' could see for themselves very clearly that they had no magical powers at all (Crowley died poor, unloved and hopelessly addicted to drugs), they still convinced themselves (and various gullible and usually wealthy followers) of the opposite.

10 THINGS TO REMEMBER

1 *Men can have multiple orgasms.*

2 *Multiple orgasms in men can be with or without ejaculation, but only a small percentage of men can learn to experience them with ejaculation.*

3 *Multiple male orgasms without ejaculation are 'brain orgasms' more than they're genital orgasms and lead directly to the state of bliss that is the aim of Tantric sex.*

4 *The first requirement for withholding ejaculation is an iron resolve, which can be helped by visualization and self-hypnosis.*

5 *The main physical techniques for withholding ejaculation include strengthening the PC muscle so as to be able to 'lock' the mechanism, together with superpanting to discharge tension and relax the cremaster muscle.*

6 *Multiple male orgasms during intercourse require the full and happy co-operation of your partner.*

7 *The vast majority of women can enjoy multiple orgasms without employing any special techniques.*

8 *The principal requirement for becoming multi-orgasmic is guilt-free, uninhibited masturbation.*

9 *A woman must be free to play with herself however she wants during intercourse (and a man must be free to do the same) because it's the owner of a body who can act with the greatest precision.*

10 *Simultaneous orgasms become simple once you've learned to control your own minds and bodies and communicate freely with one another.*

HOW TANTRIC ARE YOU NOW (MEN)?

☐ Are you practising masturbation without ejaculation most days?
☐ Are you having a session of non-ejaculatory masturbation of at least 30 minutes once a week?
☐ Are you exercising your PC muscle most days?
☐ Are you strengthening your mental resolve not to ejaculate by using visualization and self-hypnosis?
☐ Have you been able to halt ejaculation just before the PNR while having sex with your partner?
☐ Have you experienced the flood of bliss-making chemicals that accompanies a row of non-ejaculatory orgasms?
☐ Has your partner been able to enjoy her own multiple orgasms while having sex with you?
☐ Are you happy to let your partner play with herself while having intercourse with you?
☐ Do you know what triggers you can use to tip your partner over into orgasm?
☐ Can you reliably experience simultaneous orgasm with your partner when you wish?

If you answered 'yes' to between eight and ten questions you're obviously very open to Tantric sex ideas and skilled in the techniques.

If you answered 'yes' to between five and seven questions you're on your way but you have quite a bit of experimenting and practising to do.

If you couldn't answer 'yes' to more than four questions, read the chapter again and really get down to training your mind and your body. It's the most fun you'll ever have learning new things.

HOW TANTRIC ARE YOU NOW (WOMEN)?

☐ Are you happy about having a partner who masturbates frequently, either alone or with you?

☐ Are you happy about having a partner who quite often doesn't ejaculate while having sex with you?

☐ Do you enjoy taking your partner to successive peaks of non-ejaculatory excitement?

☐ Are you happy to be having more sex than you used to?

☐ Are you exercising your PC muscle most days?

☐ Are you happily enjoying uninhibited masturbation for pleasure and as a way of becoming multi-orgasmic?

☐ Are you enjoying multiple orgasms with your partner?

☐ During intercourse, can you increase your excitement at will using such techniques as self-stimulation and fantasy?

☐ Do you know what triggers you can use to tip your partner over into orgasm?

☐ Can you reliably experience simultaneous orgasm with your partner when you wish?

If you answered 'yes' to between eight and ten questions you're obviously very open to Tantric sex ideas and skilled in the techniques.

If you answered 'yes' to between five and seven questions you're on your way but you have quite a bit of experimenting and practising to do.

If you couldn't answer 'yes' to more than four questions, read the chapter again and really get down to training your mind and your body. It's the most fun you'll ever have learning new things.

9

Adhorata

In this chapter you will learn:
- *how to stimulate the male prostate*
- *how to excite your partner with analingus*
- *how to enjoy anal sex.*

> *Never should the Tantrika think in terms of pure or*
> *impure...of suitable for lovemaking or unsuitable for*
> *lovemaking. By doing so the Tantrika is cursed and will*
> *lose all magic powers.*
>
> The *Chandamaharosana Tantra*

Adhorata is one of the most powerful supplementary arousal
techniques for men and women who are open to it. It redoubles
stimulation of key sensory pathways. In women, it can stimulate
the G-spot. In men, it causes the stimulation of the 'P-spot' – the
prostate gland. As we saw in Chapter 2, in both sexes it *may*
stimulate the 'coccygeal body', a knot of blood vessels at the base
of the spine whose function is unclear to Western science but
known to Tantrikas as the '*Kundalini* gland'. It also has extremely
powerful psychological effects. The Western name for it is anal sex.

It may be you already enjoy anal sex. It may be you've tried it but
didn't enjoy it. It may be you are curious but have never tried it. It
may be you are revolted by the idea. If you're not already enjoying
anal sex, my suggestion is that you read this chapter with an open
mind before deciding.

If you're curious and want to explore new sensations, you don't have to go the whole way all at once. As we'll see in a moment, you can begin simply by stimulating the anal area externally. If that goes well, you can move on, another day, to penetration of the anal canal by a fingertip or sex toy. The final stage, when you're ready, is penetration of the rectum by a finger or fingers, by a sex toy, or by a *lingam*. There's no rush.

Everything is holy

Many people object to anal play on the grounds that it's 'dirty', both literally and morally. I'll be dealing with the anatomy of anal sex in detail in a moment but, in fact, there's no reason it has to be at all messy. Don't forget that, in Tantra, everything about the body is holy.

As regards the moral argument that anal sex is 'unnatural' and therefore wrong, many of the things human beings do are unnatural. Indeed, being unnatural is what distinguishes humans from other animals. All other species behave 'naturally' because they have no choice. Only we can behave unnaturally and it's vital that we do. Having sex without the possibility of ever getting pregnant is unnatural. Cooking is unnatural. Wearing clothes is unnatural. Shaving is unnatural. The list is endless. Whether or not something is unnatural is irrelevant in moral terms.

So let's look at what's positive about anal sex. The anal area is served by the pudendal nerve. That's the same nerve that also serves the *yonimani* (clitoris) and the *lingam*, the perineum and the scrotum, and the bulbospongiosus and ischiocavernosus muscles around the penis/vulva. In other words, stimulating the anal area sends signals along the same pathway as stimulating the *lingam* or the *yonimani*. Stimulating the anal area at the same time as the *lingam/yonimani* intensifies the signals. And other nerves are involved, too, as we'll see in a moment. So if you work on the *lingam/yonimani* and the anal area together you magnify the effect. Quite naturally.

There's also an important psychological aspect. Anal intercourse is the ultimate expression of opening yourself up, not only to your partner but to the whole universe. And, of course, a man can also be penetrated by a woman, who thus takes the role of the active goddess about as far as it can go. All of that is important in Tantric terms. But the real key to *adhorata* for Tantrikas is *Kundalini*.

As we've already seen, *Kundalini* in Tantric belief is the coiled 'serpent power' that lies 'asleep' at the base of the spine. It's absolutely fundamental to the whole philosophy of Tantra. One of the ways to arouse *Kundalini* it to have sexual intercourse. That energy can then be used to reach an altered state of consciousness. However, the route that gets closest to the 'sleeping serpent', and therefore has the most powerful effect, is not the vagina but the rectum.

Of course, the serpent is just a tool for visualization. You may or may not accept the traditional Tantric explanation of the movement of energy in the body. But what counts is that, provided you're positive about the whole concept, *adhorata works*. It introduces a new dimension and takes sexual sensation to a new level.

For heterosexual couples, there can be four different experiences of anal sex:

▶ *Shakti being done by Shiva. The response of women to anal sex is extremely varied. Toni Bentley wrote a whole memoir about it, called* The Surrender, *in which she described anal sex as an experience of God, as a way of exorcising trauma, and as preferable to vaginal sex. At the opposite end of the spectrum are women who hate it (or assume they would hate it which, in reality, they might not). In the middle are women who get excited mostly because their partners get excited. But 'surrender' is what captures the Tantric aspect because there is, indeed, a sense of opening up not only to a partner but also to the cosmos.*

▶ *Shiva doing Shakti. By contrast, just about every man would like to at least try penetrating the anus of his partner with his lingam. There are several reasons. It's breaking a taboo (which is a Tantric thing to do), providing the thrill of doing something that's 'naughty' or 'forbidden' or even, in some places, illegal. Then there's the challenge of overcoming the resistance of the exterior sphincter and the tightness of the canal. Another Tantric aspect is knowing that your partner is giving everything in the quest for oneness.*

▶ **Shiva being done by Shakti.** *Men who are open to the idea generally love being penetrated anally during sex. The opening of the anal sphincters, first with one finger, then two, three and four, raises the level of excitement enormously. And, deep inside, the prostate is the key to longer ejaculations. But, as with women, the feeling of being open to the universe is very Tantric.*

▶ **Shakti doing Shiva.** *A woman can only penetrate a man with a finger or fingers or with a sex toy. Whichever she chooses she won't, unlike a man penetrating a woman, derive any direct physical pleasure. The pleasure is all psychological. But it's not just a matter of giving her man sensations of incredible intensity. It's also about dominating, just like the Tantric goddess Kali.*

Now for the anatomy lesson.

The anatomy and the ecstasy

Most people think the anus is that little striated ring of muscle but, in fact, the anus is the hole. The ring of muscle is the external sphincter, one of a pair at either end of the anal canal. The exterior sphincter is under the control of the central nervous system and can therefore be consciously contracted and relaxed. The internal sphincter, on the other hand, is under the control of the autonomic nervous system and can't be consciously manipulated. Between the two lies the smooth tube of the anal canal, measuring about 2.5 cm (1″). No waste matter is ever left in the anal canal.

Beyond the internal sphincter lies the rectum and understanding how it functions is of key importance in pleasurable, embarrassment-free anal sex. Waste matter doesn't accumulate steadily in the rectum. Rather, it moves into the rectum from the colon at intervals and, quite often, you can feel when that's happening. After a bowel movement, the rectum will be empty and will remain empty for some time. How long is very much a personal matter but that's the 'window of opportunity' for really deep anal penetration. You need to know your body. Given that the rectum is about 20 cm (8″) long, and lies beyond the anal canal, the *lingam* of the average man can never penetrate any further.

Both men and women have prostate glands and they're in not dissimilar positions. A man's surrounds the urethra, below the bladder, and can be felt by inserting a forefinger into the rectum, about as far as it will go, and then bending it towards the pubic hair. A woman has a vagina between her rectum and her urethra, so that her prostate can be felt by inserting a finger into the vagina, not as deeply as for a man, and then curling it towards the pubic hair (see Chapter 7 for more detail). Anal penetration of a man will therefore stimulate the prostate directly. A woman's prostate can also be stimulated by a penis in the rectum but the effect is dissipated by the vagina in between. Anal penetration therefore has a more powerful effect on a man's prostate than on a woman's.

There is one other organ that may be stimulated by anal sex in both men and women. To Western science it's known as Luschka's coccygeal body, or simply the coccygeal body, and to Tantrics as the *Kundalini* gland. It's actually a dense mass of interweaving and interlocking bloods vessels that lie between the rectum and the tailbone. In other words, it can be stimulated via the rectum by pressing in the opposite direction from the prostate. According to many Tantrikas, it's this that gives anal sex its special quality in both men and women. Western science still knows very little about the coccygeal body, even though it was first described in 1860, but experiments with rats suggest it may be linked to the creation of blood cells and have an impact on dopamine, adrenaline and noradrenaline (norepinephrine). When dopamine gets into the frontal lobe of the brain it produces a feeling of bliss (and also dulls pain) so the *Kundalini gland* is a plausible explanation for some of the pleasure of anal sex (for more on *Kundalini* see Chapter 2).

But the main pleasure undoubtedly comes from the prolific nerve fibres. The pudendal nerve has already been mentioned (see p. 192). In addition, distension of the wall of the rectum sends nerve impulses to the sacral plexus along the posterior femoral cutaneous nerves. And, according to Rita Valentino of the University of Pennsylvania, the vagus nerve conveys both the sensations of genital arousal and colonic distention back to an area of the hindbrain known as the nucleus of Barrington, which in turn connects with the brain's 'pleasure pathway'. So there are direct nerve pathways as well as opportunities for a 'mingling' of signals that could make simultaneous anal sex and genital stimulation mutually reinforcing.

Before you start

Before you get going with *adhorata* there are a few issues to be sorted out. They can make the whole thing sound rather intimidating. But if you just follow the advice you won't have a problem.

LUBRICATION

Unlike the vagina, the rectum and anal canal produce no natural lubricant. Artificial lubricant is, therefore, absolutely *essential*. Never attempt anal sex of any kind without it, or the result will be pain rather than pleasure. And it's not just a question of avoiding pain there and then. Without lubrication it's quite possible to tear the lining of the anal canal and rectum which could then develop into an abscess.

If you already use a lubricant then the same one will also work in the anal canal and rectum, but many couples prefer something thicker than usual. There are lubricants made expressly for the purpose. Some couples favour a water-based gel, others like silicone-based lubricants because they remain slippery for an extremely long time (lubricants are dealt with in more detail in Chapter 5). Saliva is not enough. Get this right because, if you don't, at best you'll be put off ever doing it again, at worst there may be a visit to the hospital.

BIRTH CONTROL, SEXUAL HEALTH AND CONDOMS

Why, you might ask, do you need to consider birth control for anal sex? Well, in the first place it's unlikely to be *only* anal sex. Secondly, it's quite possible for any semen emitted to get, one way or another, into the vagina. So if you need some form of birth control for vaginal sex, then you should continue it for anal sex.

As regards sexual health, a variety of diseases can be transmitted by anal sex (and transmitted fairly easily), including HIV/AIDS, chlamydia, hepatitis, herpes, syphilis, gonorrhoea and genital warts. My advice would be not to have anal sex with someone unless you're 100 per cent certain they're not carrying any disease that could be transmitted to you. If you are 100 per cent certain, then a condom becomes optional on health grounds. If you're only 99 per cent certain or less and intend to ignore my advice then you *must* use a condom.

The other major piece of health advice is that anything that has been inside the anal canal or rectum must be dealt with appropriately:

- ▶ Condom – *whether used on the* lingam *or on a sex toy, a condom must be discarded and replaced by a new one for vaginal sex.*
- ▶ Sex toys – *must be washed or cleaned in accordance with the maker's instructions before being used for anything else, but it's better if you keep anal toys separate (for more on anal toys see below).*
- ▶ Lingam – *must be washed after anal penetration; on no account should the unwashed* lingam *come into contact with*

the vagina, vulva or mouth. (For how to deal with this pause in the proceedings see below.)

▶ **Anal area** – *it's also sensible for the person whose anus was penetrated to wash the anal area before moving on to other things.*

▶ **Finger or fingers** – *wash (it's a good idea to have one hand as your 'anal hand' so you don't get confused about what's been where – and make sure the nails are short and filed smooth).*

RELAXATION

One of the keys to enjoyable *adhorata* is relaxation. If the anal sphincters are constricted it will be difficult for anything the size of a *lingam* to get inside.

If you, the woman, feel tense about anal sex there are several things you can do:

▶ *Discuss your concerns with your partner.*
▶ *Agree that your partner will stop if you're finding it painful.*
▶ *Repeatedly visualize having enjoyable anal sex.*

When visualizing, 'see' your anus relaxed and opening up for your partner. You could even use the trance technique that's described in Chapter 7. Remember that the external sphincter is under conscious control. You can't exactly open it, as you open your mouth, but you can do the opposite of constrict it. As regards the internal sphincter, just relaxing generally will make it easier for your partner's *lingam* to pass through. Don't worry about the sphincter being used 'in reverse' – it's perfectly safe.

Exploring on your own

Before attempting *adhorata* with someone else it's best to explore your own body first. Choose a time soon after a bowel movement so the rectum will be empty.

To begin with, try caressing your own anal area using your 'anal hand' (see opposite). Probably not very exciting. As you'll discover, anal stimulation can be very powerful but only once your genitals are already aroused. So let's try again. Arouse yourself in your usual way and *then* stimulate your anal area with a well-lubricated finger. Now push it just a *little* way inside (fingernail well trimmed). There will be some resistance but not much. The tip of your finger will now be in the anal canal and it will feel very smooth and clean to the touch. In other words, if you confine your explorations to the tip of your first finger no deeper than the first joint you can't go wrong.

Take your time and remember to keep up some genital stimulation from time to time *with the other hand*. Try turning your finger in the anal canal like a key in a lock, then sliding it very slowly in and out. Which feels best?

The next stage is to penetrate further. Just beyond the depth of one finger joint, you'll encounter a second resistance. This is the interior sphincter muscle. You have no direct control over it and can't consciously relax it. However, provided you feel relaxed in general you should be able to ease your finger through it. You will now be in the rectum. Assuming you've recently has a bowel movement you won't encounter any waste matter, or only a little bit.

The nerves of the anal area are designed to respond to stretching so you'll probably find the sensation of the anus opening more arousing than other movements. Therefore, if the stimulation is going well, try using your thumb instead of a finger, then two fingers, then three (always with plenty of lubricant) to enlarge the opening.

The prostate

If you're a man, you'll probably want to locate and experiment with your prostate which is a very vital part of your sexual apparatus. One of its roles is to contribute prostatic fluid to the semen, and the more it can be encouraged to produce, the longer ejaculation can continue (if that's what you want). What's more, its contractions contribute to the pleasurable feelings of orgasm, via the hypogastric nerve. Consequently, the prostate is one of the keys to great sex.

The prostate encircles the urethra, like a tiny doughnut, well inside the body just below the bladder. As it lies about 5.5 cm (2.25″) from the anus, you'll have to insert your finger up to the second joint, with the pad facing towards your navel. Now press on the wall of the rectum. Don't curl your finger. You'll know if you're on the prostate because it feels quite distinct and is about the size of a grape (although it could be much larger if you're past 50). If you can't identify it as something quite separate from the surrounding tissue, then you're not on it. The final test is to keep your finger there while you masturbate to ejaculation. You'll feel the prostate contract several times. Don't confuse the contractions with the pulsation of the blood vessel there. You'll know the difference by the fact that the blood keeps on pumping once the ejaculation is over, although less forcefully, whereas the prostate doesn't.

Stimulation of the prostate should feel very nice and will, if continued, cause some liquid to be expelled from the penis. Men over 50, however, might not feel very much from direct prostate stimulation, although the anal penetration should continue to be exciting.

Insight

Unlike masturbation, anal pleasure is something that has to be cultivated. It's more subtle than genital stimulation because it's more of an adjunct, rather like salt added to food. No one would want to eat salt on its own, but once you've experienced salt on your food you wouldn't want to have dinner without it. So it is with anal penetration. It makes the effect of the main dish (stimulation of *lingam/ yoni/yonimani*) all the more vivid. Once you're starting to enjoy yourself on your own, it's time to involve your partner, who, hopefully, has also been experimenting alone.

Doing it well

Men and women who are used to anal sex may not need much 'warming up' but newcomers or those who make anal play only a rare ingredient in their lovemaking will need plenty of time to get prepared. Don't rush. There's a huge difference between good anal sex and bad anal sex and much of the difference is to do with taking time. Linger over *nyasa* and *auparishtaka*. What comes next? I'd suggest analingus.

ANALINGUS

Analingus, or rimming, means stimulating your partner's anal area with your tongue. Of course, your partner must have had a bath or shower immediately beforehand.

Have a go (Shakti by Shiva)
- ▶ Step 1: *While performing* auparishtaka *on your partner's vulva, and only when she's aroused, make a few long licks from end to end, including the anal area.*
- ▶ Step 2: *If Step 1 was popular, spend a little time running the tip of your tongue round and round the external sphincter.*
- ▶ Step 3: *Continue* auparishtaka, *now including the anal area.*

ANAL PENETRATION (SHAKTI BY SHIVA)

After analingus, my advice would be to have vaginal sex for a few minutes to get Shakti really aroused. While that's going on, place the well-lubricated forefinger of your 'anal hand' on Shakti's sphincter, circle it and then slide it gently inside. You'll be able to feel your *lingam* in her *yoni*, which is exciting for both of you. If you can give your partner an orgasm without ejaculating yourself that would be perfect. Now you're both ready for anal penetration with the *lingam*.

Have a go

▶ **Step 1:** *The first consideration is position. Given that the anus and the opening of the vagina are very close together, it's theoretically possible to have anal sex in almost any position in which you enjoy vaginal sex. In reality, the fact that the vagina is very easy to get into, even when you can't see it, makes a considerable difference. As beginners I suggest you start with a position not described in either the* Kama Sutra *or the* Ananga Ranga *and which does not have, as far as I'm aware, a Sanskrit name. Shakti kneels on the bed, thighs comfortably apart, resting her shoulders and head on a pillow. This exposes the anus and puts it at the right height and angle for you. (For more on positions, see Chapter 10.) It also mimics the lordosis or 'presenting' behaviour of mammals such as the cat, creating a really primeval mindset.*

▶ **Step 2:** *Don't go for penetration with the* lingam *straight away. There's still a bit more preparation to do. You should now circle the anus with a lubricated finger. Your partner should find that very enjoyable. If so, gently insert the forefinger (nail closely trimmed) of your 'anal hand' as far as the first joint. (As an alternative to fingers you might prefer a sex toy – see p. 207.) The sensation of the anus opening may feel confusing at first, so give your partner plenty of time to get used to it. If all goes well, the next stage is to replace your forefinger with your thumb (nail well trimmed), again using plenty of lubrication. From a thumb you might progress to two fingers, the tips pressed close together, and then to three. (Note that while it's easy to open the anus with the pad of one finger, using two or more fingers brings the nails into play so great care must be taken.) At every opportunity add more lubricant so that it lines the anal canal and rectum. And use your 'non-anal hand' to caress her buttocks or tantalize her* yonimani.

▶ **Step 3:** *When you see that Shakti's sphincter is relaxing, prepare your* lingam. *It may well be that while you've been giving all your attention to your partner your erection has gone down somewhat. That's no problem because as you're coating your* lingam *with lubricant (using your 'non-anal hand') so it will become hard again.*

▶ **Step 4:** *It's a curious feature of the external sphincter that, once relaxed, the anus doesn't immediately close up when fingers (or a sex toy) are withdrawn. You'll have a second or two – but not much more – to take advantage of the open anus to insert your* lingam. *However, if you miss that moment don't worry. As long as your partner is relaxed, and as long as you have a fairly hard erection, you'll still be able to ease your lubricated* lingam *a little way inside. In the case that your partner is willing but her external sphincter clamps her anus resolutely shut, see the Insight on p. 204.*

▶ **Step 5:** *Once inside the anal canal, gently push a little further until your glans is out of sight and then stop. Let Shakti get used to the sensations before doing anything else. This is important because it's going to take a minute or two for her body to adjust.*

▶ **Step 6:** *You now have various options and, of course, it all depends on Shakti. You could slowly ease your* lingam *all the way and then make some gentle backwards and forwards movements. You could remain half way. You could reach round with your 'non-anal hand' and stimulate her clitoris (unless she thinks it's already had enough stimulation). You could insert the forefinger of your 'non-anal hand' into her vagina and tickle her G-spot (see Chapter 7) or feel yourself inside her rectum. You can caress her buttocks and bite her neck... And, of course, Shakti may do some moving herself. Note that some women quite like the feeling of the* lingam *being taken out and reinserted, while others aren't very keen at all on that initial sensation of the* lingam *going in. So Shakti needs to be able to say what she likes and dislikes without embarrassment or anxiety.*

▶ **Step 7:** *Hopefully, Shakti will have an orgasm from the combined effects of anal penetration and the other things you're doing. Maybe not. What about you? I'd suggest you utilize the control techniques you learned in the previous chapter in order to withhold ejaculation. Semen in the rectum is messy and can cause uncomfortable irritation which might put your partner off doing it again. If you're wearing a condom those considerations won't apply, but if you are* *going to ejaculate, Shakti will almost certainly find it much more exciting in the vagina.*

▶ **Step 8:** *You, Shiva, must now go and wash. It's a good idea for Shakti to do the same. So a shower together would be an ideal solution.*

▶ **Step 9:** *Having enjoyed your interlude in the shower you can now resume lovemaking.*

Insight

If you're having a problem getting your lingam into the anal canal, a trick is to insert the tip of your forefinger ('anal hand' remember!) into Shakti's anus, or to ask her to insert the tip of her own forefinger. You can then use that like a shoehorn to keep you on target and stop you slipping away into the vagina.

TIPS FOR SHAKTIS

If you've never experienced *adhorata* before, you may have the feeling that you are going, or want to go, to the toilet. That's normal to begin with because that's how your body has always reacted up till now. So you may not enjoy it very much the first time (especially not if it's also the first time for your partner). As I've said, it's something of an acquired taste and not as immediately exciting as clitoral or vaginal stimulation. And it requires considerable skill from your partner. However, it will become more exciting as your body gets used to the new sensations. So you really need to have a few sessions before you can make a definitive judgement. Some experienced women find it quite mind-blowing.

Make sure plenty of lubricant is being used. No lubricant, no anal penetration. There's no reason you shouldn't slap some on yourself, around the opening, inside and on his *lingam*.

In the position described, you can reach behind and separate your buttocks if your partner is having a problem – he can then use the forefinger of his 'anal hand' as a shoehorn, and his other hand to guide his *lingam* in.

Don't be backward about saying what you don't like (but not in a critical way).

Don't be embarrassed about saying what you do like. (In my focus groups, men often say they never know if their partners are enjoying the anal sex or not, because nothing is said.)

You can take charge of movement if you like. Tell your partner to stay still while you explore the sensations created by moving backwards and forwards.

The whole point of *adhorata* is to arouse *Kundalini* and open yourself to a state of oneness with your partner and, if you wish, the entire universe. This is about as open as you can get, so take the opportunity to revel in that sensation and, with your head on the pillow and your eyes closed, you have the perfect set-up for 'sexual meditation'.

Insight

While you, Shakti, are being anally penetrated by your partner's lingam you might find it exciting to insert a finger into your vagina so you can feel what's going on through the thin wall that separates it from your rectum.

ANAL PENETRATION (SHIVA BY SHAKTI)

There are various ways in which you, Shakti, can penetrate your man anally. I'm going to describe one particularly good way which is almost guaranteed to produce a cosmic experience, or at least give your partner the best physical sex he's ever had. Afterwards, don't touch your vulva with the same fingers until they've been washed.

Warning: Don't try to penetrate your man anally with a finger if you have long, sharp or ragged nails. That's potentially dangerous. If long nails are important to you, use a sex toy instead (see p. 207).

Have a go

▶ **Step 1:** *Make love in the* Uttana-bandha *(missionary-type) position with a couple of pillows under your buttocks so Shiva can penetrate your vagina while* squatting *between your thighs (for more on positions see Chapter 10).*

▶ **Step 2:** *When Shiva is nicely excited but not too close to ejaculation (otherwise this will send him straight over the edge), reach under his buttocks and place a* lubricated *forefinger (nail trimmed and filed smooth) on his anus. That should already do quite a lot.*

▶ **Step 3:** *Run your lubricated finger round and round the sphincter and then slowly push it in up to about the first joint. Watch his eyes roll upwards.*

▶ **Step 4:** *Try gently turning your finger. The lining of the anal canal is extremely smooth and this should give him a very agreeable sensation.*

▶ **Step 5:** *If all is going well, gently push in a little further.*

▶ **Step 6:** *Withdraw your finger, add more lubricant to your first and middle fingers, and insert the two pressed tightly together.*

▶ **Step 7:** *For even more sensation try three and then four fingers, always with plenty of lubrication. Experiment gently. Try rotating your hand as well as moving slowly in and out. Most men will probably be happiest just with the sense of the anus being opened. Ask.*

▶ **Step 8:** *You could now try for the prostate. For how to find it, see the dedicated section on pp. 199–200. Stroke the prostate gently. Watch to see what effect you're having.*

Although anal stimulation normally magnifies genital stimulation, it is possible to overdo it, such that the whole focus moves to the anal area and rectum and Shiva's erection wanes. So this has interesting possibilities for both increasing and decreasing genital energy and controlling ejaculation.

Of course, you're doing all this while your partner is making love to you and, hopefully, giving you very nice sensations as well. So you may not be able to do these things quite as coolly as the descriptions suggest. It will be a terrific test of your partner's ejaculation control and many men will fail it the first time. No doubt his excitement will be infectious and you should be able to enjoy spectacular simultaneous orgasms.

An excellent alternative position is to make love on your side, face to face with Shiva and have him bring his upper thigh over your hip. Like this you can easily slide a finger or two into his anal canal and rectum. If you bend your own legs he can simultaneously do the same to you.

Insight

Are men who enjoy anal penetration by their female partners gay? Of course not. It isn't what you do but who you do it with. If you're only attracted to women then you're straight, no matter how excited you get by having your partner stretch your sphincter, or stroke your prostate. If you are a gay man or woman, I should stress that you can still practise Tantric sex. Some of the physical techniques may need a little adaptation here and there, but provided your aim is to reach a higher spiritual level then, in my opinion, the title 'Tantric sex' still applies.

Anal sex toys

Vibrators can create some very intense sensations in the anal canal and rectum. And if you're a bit squeamish, they get around the challenge of putting your finger inside. You could use your vaginal vibrator (see Chapter 4) in the anal canal and rectum, provided it's not too big, but it's better to buy a second vibrator specifically designed for the purpose. Once again, you don't have to buy something plastic if you don't want; you can buy anal toys in glass and even jade. Anal vibrators are narrower and shorter than standard models and usually have a wide base to stop them accidentally slipping all the way in. Apart from that, it's more hygienic to have a separate vibrator for the anal area. There's also a very special kind of anal dildo specifically designed for the prostate gland. After insertion into the rectum via the anus, the man flexes his PC muscle to press the head of the dildo against the gland and massage it. As a result, the gland produces an increased quantity of prostatic fluid, leading to longer and more satisfying ejaculations. This is something a man can do while masturbating or just prior to beginning a Tantric sex session.

> **Warning:** It's a good idea to put a condom over your anal toy. When the session is over you only need to peel off the condom and dispose of it. But it's still a good idea to rinse the toy too.

PRACTISING ON YOUR OWN

As always, it's a good idea to practise new techniques on yourself before trying them out with your partner.

Have a go
▶ **Step 1:** *Excite yourself in your usual way.*
▶ **Step 2:** *Apply plenty of lubricant to your anus and to the vibrator, switch on and insert it a short distance.*
▶ **Step 3:** *As you get used to the sensations so you can ease it further inside if you want or you can just keep it at the entrance where most of the nerve endings are.*
▶ **Step 4:** *Experiment with the effects of changing the balance between anal and genital stimulation. Does anal stimulation add to sensation in the genitals or diminish it?*

USING AN ANAL VIBRATOR DURING INTERCOURSE

A particularly exciting way of using an anal vibrator is to slip it into your partner's rectum during intercourse.

Have a go (Shiva to Shakti)
▶ **Step 1:** *Make love in a rear entry position.*
▶ **Step 2:** *At a suitable moment, Shiva should apply lubricant to Shakti's anus and to the vibrator.*
▶ **Step 3:** *Switch on the vibrator, tease Shakti's sphincter with it and gently slip it inside. Check that she's happy.*

► **Step 4:** *Continue making love. Shakti will additionally feel the vibrations throughout her pubic area and you'll feel them along your* lingam. *It will be intensely exciting for both of you.*

Have a go (Shakti to Shiva)
The other way of using an anal vibrator during intercourse is for Shakti to slip it into the Shiva's rectum.

► **Step 1:** *Make love in a man-on-top position.*
► **Step 2:** *At a suitable moment, Shakti should apply lubricant to Shiva's anus and to the vibrator.*
► **Step 3:** *Switch on the vibrator, tease Shiva's sphincter with it and gently slip it inside. Check that he's happy.*
► **Step 4:** *Continue making love. Shiva will additionally feel the vibrations throughout his groin and you, Shakti, will pick them up from his* lingam *and sense them throughout your* yoni.

10 THINGS TO REMEMBER

1 *Anal stimulation magnifies genital stimulation and takes sex to a new level, involving the pudendal, vagus and femoral cutaneous nerves and directly arousing* Kundalini.

2 *If you've not yet experienced anal sex, try to keep an open mind.*

3 *Tantra considers everything about the body to be holy, including the anal canal and rectum.*

4 *The anal canal is always empty and there are periods when the rectum is also empty.*

5 *Don't have anal sex with someone unless you're 100 per cent certain they have no diseases they could transmit to you.*

6 *Artificial lubrication is absolutely essential for anal stimulation of any kind – no lubricant, no anal sex.*

7 *Spend plenty of time on anal foreplay to get the sphincters relaxed.*

8 *If you're having a problem getting your* lingam *into the anal canal, you can use a fingertip to 'shoehorn' it in.*

9 *Most men will enjoy being anally penetrated by their partner's fingers during sex.*

10 *Anal vibrators can create very intense sensations.*

HOW TANTRIC ARE YOU NOW?

- ☐ Have you tried stimulating your own anal area?
- ☐ Have you explored inside your anal canal and rectum (using plenty of lubricant on your finger)?
- ☐ Have you explored your own/partner's prostate gland?
- ☐ Have you had a go at analingus?
- ☐ Have you tried stimulating your partner's anal area during sex?
- ☐ Have you slipped a finger into your partner's anal canal and rectum during sex?
- ☐ Has the *lingam* been in the anal canal?
- ☐ Has the *lingam* been in the rectum?
- ☐ Have you had/caused an orgasm during anal sex?
- ☐ Have you tried any anal sex toys?

If you answered 'yes' to between eight and ten questions you're obviously very open to Tantric sex ideas and have worked hard on acquiring the skills.

If you answered 'yes' to between five and seven questions you're on your way but you have quite a bit of experimenting and practising to do.

If you couldn't answer 'yes' to more than four questions, maybe you're thinking that *adhorata* just isn't for you. In that case, read the chapter again, mull it over and, perhaps, try out a few little things on your own. Remember that Tantric sex is all about overcoming inhibitions, overthrowing taboos, the holiness of everything about the body and, of course, having mind-altering sensations.

10

Tantric positions

In this chapter you will learn:
- *why women should get on top*
- *how to 'speak' the 'secret language'*
- *the best positions for long, meditative* maithuna
- *the best positions for G-spot stimulation*
- *the best positions for* adhorata.

> *Shiva without Shakti is a corpse.*
>
> Tantric saying

In Tantric (and Hindu) belief, the Divine Consciousness has always existed and will always exist. It has no beginning and no end. According to the **Vedas**, there was neither what is nor what is not. The darkness was hidden in darkness. But in that infinite peace, the ONE was breathing by its own power. And in the ONE, love arose.

The ONE, pictured as a male god, and often given the name Shiva, was passive. Shiva didn't do anything until, feeling lonely, he created the female, often called Shakti, to keep him company. It was the active lovemaking of Shakti, together with the power of Shiva, that created the visible universe. Hence the Tantric saying, 'Shiva without Shakti is a corpse.'

And, indeed, the two lovemaking gods who created the entire universe are often depicted in this way. In paintings and in statuettes, Shiva lies flat on his back, unmoving, while Shakti (or quite often the 'terrible goddess' Kali) sits astride him, writhing and grinding, extracting his energy so that she can power Creation. Sometimes the god is depicted lying on an actual corpse, signifying his alter ego, in a state beyond time and space when he was alone as the ONE.

So what does all this have to do with lovemaking positions?

What makes a position Tantric?

Tantrikas believe that when they make love they're copying Shiva and Shakti and taking part in the 'cosmic dance', playing a role, as it were, in the maintenance of Creation. The whole visible universe is, after all, nothing more than the vibrations set up by the lovemaking deities. Inspired by the legend of Shiva and Shakti, they believe that the most Tantric positions or *asanas* are those in which:

▶ *the woman is on top*
▶ *the woman does the moving*
▶ *the man stays still*
▶ *special energy patterns are created.*

In fact, I shall argue that various other kinds of positions can fulfil the Tantric aim of arousing *Kundalini* (sexual energy) just as well or even better. But if there's little physical movement in the most Tantric positions, that certainly doesn't mean there's no excitement at all because there's always the 'secret language'.

The secret language

Shiva and Shakti sit or lie together without visibly moving. And yet they're almost delirious with pleasure because they're 'speaking' to one another in the 'secret language'. Invisibly, Shakti contracts her vaginal muscles to squeeze and stroke the *lingam* inside her, creating a sensation similar to a man's thrusting.

Here is what the fourteenth/fifteenth century Indian sex manual, the *Ananga Ranga* (translated 1873), had to say on the subject:

> *At all times of enjoying Purushayita [woman-on-top positions] the wife will remember that without an especial exertion of will on her part, the husband's pleasure will not be perfect. To this end she must ever strive to close and constrict the Yoni until it holds the Linga, as with a finger, opening and shutting at her pleasure, and finally, acting as the hand of the Gopala-girl, who milks the cow. This can be learned only by long practice, and especially by throwing the will into the part to be affected, even as men endeavour to sharpen their hearing, and their sense of touch. While so doing, she will mentally repeat 'Kamadeva! Kamadeva!' in order that a blessing may rest upon the undertaking... Her husband will then value her above all women, nor would he exchange her for the most beautiful Rani (queen) in the three worlds.*

Sir Richard Burton, the Victorian explorer, sexologist and co-translator of the *Ananga Ranga* as well as the *Kama Sutra*, added the following footnote:

> *Amongst some races the constrictor vaginae muscles are abnormally developed. In Abyssinia, for instance, a woman can so exert them as to cause pain to a man, and, when sitting upon his thighs, she can induce the orgasm without moving any other part of her person... All women have more or less the power, but they wholly neglect it...*

No doubt, Burton, who led a very full life, was writing from personal experience. So what do you, the woman, do to develop Burton's 'abnormal' muscles and move your *yoni* in the same way that the hand of the 'Gopala-girl' milks a cow? We're talking about being able to control individually all the muscles that surround the *yoni*, not just in two blocks as we did in Chapter 8.

Have a go
▶ **Step 1:** *Slide a lubricated finger into the entrance of your* yoni *and try to grip it.*

- ▶ **Step 2:** *Now try to pull it inside.*
- ▶ **Step 3:** *Repeat steps 1 and 2 until you've identified the different muscular action involved in gripping and in pulling.*
- ▶ **Step 4:** *Insert a lubricated dildo into the yoni and try gripping it, first only with the muscles at the entrance to the yoni and then, bit by bit, contracting the muscles all the way up to the cervix.*
- ▶ **Step 5:** *Relax the muscles bit by bit, beginning at the cervix and ending at the entrance.*
- ▶ **Step 6:** *Repeat step 4, then again relax the muscles but this time beginning at the entrance and working along to the cervix.*
- ▶ **Step 7:** *Make the dildo move in and out by muscular action of the yoni.*
- ▶ **Step 8:** *Make the part of the dildo that's sticking out go round and round in circles by muscular action of the yoni.*
- ▶ **Step 9:** *Practise with a lingam and ask your partner to tell you where and how much he feels the sensations.*
- ▶ **Step 10:** *You know you've succeeded when your partner reports it's like being stroked, from one end of the lingam to the other.*

Like the Tantrikas of old you can also use an 'egg' for some of the exercises (nowadays stainless steel eggs or 'vaginal dumbbells' from sex shops are preferred to stones). Of course, you don't have to practise all ten steps at once. Keep on with the PC exercises in Chapter 8 and gradually increase your prowess in the secret language over the next few weeks.

Shiva can also 'reply' in the secret language by flexing his lingam inside the yoni, which his Shakti will be able to feel and enjoy. For this, he too needs to exercise his PC muscle in the way described in Chapter 8.

SOME OTHER CONSIDERATIONS

Every position has its own special qualities, combining different aspects of Tantric ritual.

Breathing
In Chapter 4 we looked at the various ways of breathing. The positions best suited to co-ordinating inhalation, exhalation and

the movement of *prana* include *yab yum*, *mula bandha* (time your breathing to the up and down movement), *yoni asana* and *parshva piditaka*, all of which are described below.

Mantras

You might like to intone your mantras prior to intercourse or, if you like, you can also intone them during intercourse. *OM* works well (see Chapter 4) especially with *mula bandha*. Intone 'aah' as you sit up, 'oh' as you remain upright for a moment, and 'ong' as you lower yourselves down and repose a while before beginning all over again.

Meeting of eyes

They say the eyes are the windows on the soul and, of course, it's true. Tantrikas talk of 'melting through the gaze' which means achieving total union like two pats of liquefying butter. Static face-to-face positions such as *yab yum* and *yoni asana* are perfect for this. Try looking, unblinking, into one another's eyes for two minutes. There's a profound sense of making contact with something that is apart from the physical body. Is it real or is it an illusion? You can also stare at one another's 'third eyes' at the *Ajna* chakra (see Chapter 2).

Alternatively, when oneness with the whole universe is your goal, you'll want to look away, fixing your gaze on a candle, a star or, perhaps, an image generated by your own mind.

ENERGY CIRCULATION

As we saw in Chapter 2, arousing *Kundalini* and circulating energy are important aspects of Tantric sex and, with that in mind, some of the positions (for example, the X postures on p. 219) need to be copied quite precisely.

ALTERED STATES OF CONSCIOUSNESS

Position will have an effect on your state of consciousness. If you're mainly interested in increasing your sense of oneness with your partner, of trying to make contact with your partner's soul, of striving to feel that you have one body and one mind between you, then you need to choose positions such as *vinaka-tiryak-bandha* that put you very close together, face to face, with your eyes meeting. If, on the other hand, your aim is to experience a sense of oneness with the whole of Creation then you need to choose positions in which your contact is at the genitals alone and in which you don't look at one another (for example, Kali-in-a-good-mood, leaning right back).

Goddess-on-top meditative positions

These positions are extremely sensual and also potentially very spiritual. It may seem, however, that they're not highly stimulating sexually and, indeed, that's the whole point. Because they're positions in which it's difficult for *lingam* and *yoni* to create much friction they're perfect for long, meditative sessions in which Shiva should be able to continue for extended periods without ejaculating. Nevertheless, the potential for sexual excitement shouldn't be underestimated when Shakti knows the 'secret language' (see p. 213).

Older men may have a problem with woman-on-top positions because the force of gravity is working against blood flow into the penis and inhibiting erection. If that's the case for you, then a possible solution is to withdraw from time to time to self-stimulate. Or you could gently tip your partner onto her back, when your erection wanes and continue like that.

YAB YUM

This is probably the most famous Tantric sex position. Shiva sits on the floor or on the bed in the lotus position, or the half-lotus, or simply with legs crossed (in which case this pose may also be known as *sukhapadma asana*). Shakti then lowers her *yoni* onto her partner's *lingam* and sits on his lap, crossing her ankles behind his back.

Like this, you can look into one another's eyes and lock yourselves together, tongue to tongue, breast to breast and, of course, *yoni* to *lingam*. With your faces close together you can breathe in harmony, co-ordinating inhalation and exhalation with rocking backwards and forwards or from side to side. It's also a classic position for energy circulation.

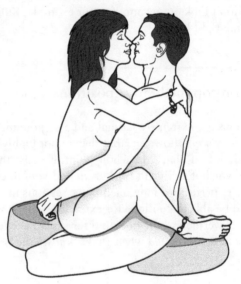

Figure 10.1 Yab yum.

MULA BANDHA

This is a development from *yab yum*. Holding one another's arms, you both slowly lean back until your heads are resting on the floor or bed and then slowly pull one another upright again. This movement creates just enough friction between *yoni* and *lingam* and should be repeated again and again to maintain a blissful excitement. As a refinement, your feet should press into the base of your partner's spine each time you both lie back.

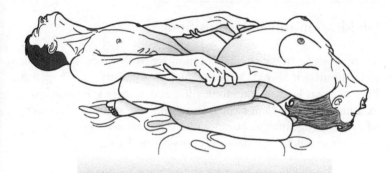

Figure 10.2 Mula bandha.

MULA BANDHA *VARIATIONS – THE X POSTURES*

In variation one, rather than repeatedly pulling one another up and down, as in *mula bandha* (above), you remain either lying motionless, flat on the floor (for a more cosmic effect) or propped up a little on cushions (so that the meeting of eyes is possible).

Variation two is slightly more complicated. Sit on the floor or bed facing one another. Shiva now puts his right leg over Shakti's left, while she puts her right leg over the Shiva's left. Shuffling towards one another, you unite *yoni* and *lingam*. You then lie back flat. To complete the posture you clasp one another's wrists in a particular way. Shakti puts her left arm under Shiva's right leg while he puts his right arm over her left leg; she puts her right arm over his left leg and he puts his left arm under her right leg. You each now turn your heads to your right, so you're facing in opposite directions – the idea is to allow you to focus on your own sensations and your vision of cosmic oneness.

Although the man's erection will gradually subside, his *lingam* is pretty much locked into the *yoni* (a *bandha* is a 'lock') and should not slip out.

Goddess-on-top active positions

In any position in which Shakti can move freely, understanding has to be intuitive if Shiva is to enjoy multiple orgasms (see Chapter 8). But once that level of communication exists, there's nothing more exciting for a man than to be taken again and again by his Shakti to the very edge of ejaculation without going over. She then becomes as much a goddess as is possible on Earth.

YONI ASANA *WITH FEET ON THE FLOOR*

Yoni asana is similar to *yab yum* except that, instead of sitting on the bed or carpet, Shiva sits on a chair or couch with his feet on the floor and Shakti sits on his thighs, facing him, with her ankles crossed behind his back. The effects are very similar to *yab yum* but if Shakti also puts *her* feet on the floor, the dynamics are completely changed. In addition to the 'secret language' and to churning, Shakti can now slide up and down the *lingam* as she pleases, causing maximum excitement.

KALI ASANA

For some Tantrikas, it's Kali not Shakti who is the supreme goddess. In the *Devimahatmya* she's described as fearsome, grotesque and demonic, with the severed heads and limbs of those she's slain hanging as ornaments on her otherwise naked body. In the *Kalika Purana* she rides a lion, has four arms and is beautiful. And in the *Sakti-samgama Tantra*, which inspires this position, she pleasures herself on the supine body of Shiva. But whichever of the traditions you follow, Kali is always her own woman (or goddess) and does as she pleases. You, the woman, must do the same. Order your man to lie flat on his back and straddle him, supporting yourself on your knees, and swallowing up his *lingam* with your *yoni*. Now, like Kali, pleasure yourself however you wish. You can churn, you can slide up and down or you can sit still and use the secret language. You can be upright or you can change the angle of your *yoni* by leaning back a little, your hands on his knees, or leaning forwards a little, your hands on his shoulders. You can unashamedly caress your own *yonimani* and breasts or you can order your partner to caress you exactly how you want. But don't forget that, if the aim is a prolonged, altered state of consciousness, your wild inclinations will have to be tempered with the utmost skill.

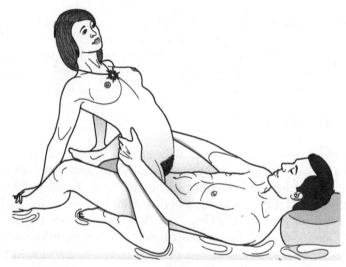

Figure 10.3 Kali asana.

PURUSHAYITA-BHRAMARA-BANDHA

This is similar to *Kali asana*, except that Shakti squats on her feet. This small change creates an enormous difference because, in contrast to *Kali asana*'s kneeling position, it allows Shakti to keep *lingam* and *yoni* in exquisite alignment as she slides up and down. Shiva must provide support by taking a buttock in each hand – this gives him some control and, at the same time, he can also tantalize Shakti's anus with his little fingers. If there's a danger of going beyond the PNR, then Shiva has only to hold Shakti still. Shakti can vary the effect by either closing her thighs to grip Shiva's *lingam* as in a vice, or opening them widely to expose her labia and *yonimani* to Shiva's eyes and caresses.

UTTHITA-UTTANA-BANDHA

Again similar to *Kali asana*, in this version you, the woman, sit cross-legged on your man. You can churn and use the secret language but to move and up and down you'll have to use your arms.

KALI'S TRAP

You, Kali, order your man to lie on his side. Take hold of his upper leg, raise it and, facing him, kneel down to straddle his lower thigh. You can now slide forwards to seize his *lingam* in your *yoni*. You can rub your *yonimani* against his upper thigh or stimulate it with your fingers.

KALI'S REVENGE

In this position, the fearsome Kali completely turns the tables on men. Order your partner to lie on his back with his knees drawn back to his chest and his calves and feet in the air. In this way his buttocks and thighs make the seat of a chair, while his calves and feet become the back of a chair. You, Kali, then have the choice of straddling the 'seat', facing your partner, or of sitting down on the 'seat' in the normal manner, facing away from your partner. Either way, penetration will not be very deep.

KALI-IN-A-GOOD-MOOD

Kali is feeling a little gentler on this occasion and willing to allow her partner a position of near equality. The man kneels and either sits on his feet or sits between his feet, whichever is most comfortable. He spreads his thighs and leans back a little, placing his hands behind him to help take the weight of his upper body. Kali now squats down onto her partner's *lingam* and while sitting on his thighs also leans back, just as he is doing, taking her weight on her arms. It's a position with a lot of subtle variations. You can both vary how much you open or close your thighs, to help control the sexual tension, and also vary how much you lean back, so you can be close and intimate or, at the other extreme, lean away to meditate on your cosmic experience.

Shiva-in-control positions

Although many gurus and books on Tantric sex teach that the Shakti-on-top static positions are the best for guaranteeing extended lovemaking, I have to disagree. Only Shiva knows precisely how close he is to the PNR so, logically, he, rather than Shakti, needs to be in control. And while the static poses do indeed make movement difficult that's not to say you can't remain perfectly still in other positions when you need to. Most of all, Tantric sex is all about an altered state of consciousness and the greater the excitement, the more easily that altered state is achieved. However, there's no need to choose between one kind of position and another. One day you can use one kind, another day another kind, and another day every kind.

DHENUKA-VYANTA-BANDHA

A woman who has developed the skill can ejaculate in just about any position, but most beginners find it easiest if they stand in this position, which is described in both the *Kama Sutra* and the *Ananga Ranga*. Both ancient texts require Shakti to bend over and place her hands on the ground in a 'cow posture', but modern Western women are unlikely to be that flexible. For considerably more enjoyment you, the woman, can simply lean forwards and support yourself on anything convenient (chair, table, tree, rock or whatever). An aggressive partner risks pushing you over but as this is Tantric sex, Shiva will be gentle and concentrate on keeping the head of his *lingam* in contact with your G-spot (see Chapter 7 if you've forgotten where it is).

LORDOSIS

This position, mentioned in the previous chapter, doesn't seem to have a Sanskrit name, so I'm calling it 'lordosis'. Lordosis is, in fact, the 'presenting' behaviour of mammals such as the cat, in which the hind quarters are raised and the spine is bent downwards like a banana. And as Shiva is, in effect, the 'lord' of the universe, so the name has a double meaning. In the West, it's often unromantically known as 'doggy'. Shakti kneels on the bed, thighs comfortably apart, and either supports herself on her arms or, better still, rests her shoulders and head on a pillow. This gives Shiva a magnificent view, making him 'lord' of all he surveys. (If you, Shakti, are embarrassed about that, you might first like to try the position out in the dark.) Shiva enters kneeling.

It's a position that allows for excellent G-spot contact and all kinds of additional stimulation. Shiva can, for example, reach around and stroke Shakti's breasts, nipples and *yonimani*. He can lean forward and nuzzle and gently bite her ears and neck. And he can run a lubricated finger around her anal area.

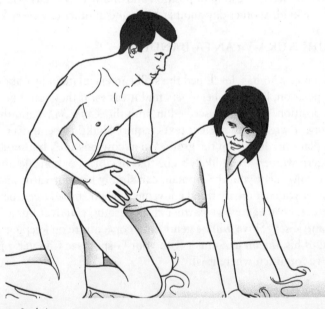

Figure 10.4 Lordosis.

For a completely different set of sensations he can also lean well back, so the *lingam* is the only point of contact, thus freeing him to meditate. As for Shakti, having opened herself up to the maximum, she too can concentrate on using the sexual energy for a cosmic experience.

> **Warning:** A disadvantage of this and other rear-entry positions is that, with vigorous movement, Shakti can get pumped full of air, which becomes very uncomfortable. It's important to stop from time to time to let the air escape.

AYBHA-VYANTA-BANDHA

In this rear-entry position, in which Shakti lies face down on the bed, the head of the *lingam* is almost guaranteed to stimulate the G-spot. But in order to get into position, it's easiest if you, the woman, begin on your hands and knees (as for lordosis above). Once the *lingam* is in the *yoni*, gradually lower yourself down. Shiva will now be sitting on your upper thighs and, because of that and the angle, his glans should be just where you want it. If not, one or two pillows under your hips should put things right. This is a position in which you should both find it easy to continue for an extended period. Shakti's excitement can be increased by placing a vibrator on the bed, touching her *yonimani* (take care that, due to the weight on it, it doesn't press to hard and hurt). Shiva can also very easily bite her neck, gently pull her hair, massage her back and buttocks and play with her anal area. So this can easily be a position in which Shiva can create a sense of oneness with Shakti or you can both concentrate on your own sensations and your visions.

TIRYAKASANA

Tiryak means 'sideways' but, in fact, only Shiva is sideways. Begin lying side by side, Shakti on Shiva's left. Shakti remains on her back, her legs open as if for the missionary position. Shiva turns onto his left side, lifting his partner's right leg over his right hip, while sliding his left leg under her left leg. In other words, Shakti's left leg is between Shiva's legs and *yoni* and *lingam* can be united. This is a comfortable position that can be maintained a long time, while allowing limited movement.

VINAKA-TIRYAK-BANDHA

In this variation on the sideways theme, with Shiva and Shakti face to face, Shiva bends his upper leg and places it over Shakti's hip. By doing so he exposes his scrotum and anal area to Shakti.

KARKATA-TIRYAK-BANDHA

Shiva and Shakti are on their sides, Shiva between Shakti's thighs, so one is under him and one over him. In other words, if you roll onto your sides from the missionary position you'll be in *karkata-tiryak-bandha*. It can be a nice position in which to take a bit of a rest but when a little more stimulation is needed, Shiva has only to raise Shakti's upper leg to see the beauty of her *yoni* and thrust.

PARSHVA PIDITAKA

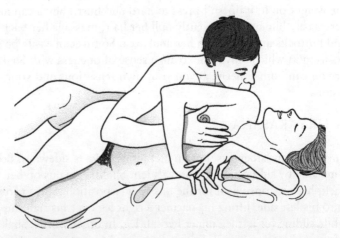

Figure 10.5 Parshva piditaka.

This is the position that, in the West, is often called 'spoons'. Shakti lies on her side, her legs a little bent. Shiva, also on his side, presses himself against her, and enters from behind. So, in effect, this is *aybha-vyanta-bandha* (see p. 225) turned sideways. In order to actually get the *lingam* into the *yoni*, Shakti may have to bend her legs rather more and Shiva may have to lift her upper leg. Once the *lingam* is inside, however, it's possible to adopt the classic 'spoon', nestling comfortably together.

VESHTITA ASANA

Shakti, on her back and with a pillow under her buttocks, crosses her ankles and places her feet against Shiva's chest. This really opens the *yoni* but, at the same time, tantalizes the squatting Shiva by preventing him from thrusting too deeply.

Squatting

In Tantric sex, whenever appropriate, Shiva squats rather than kneels, and kneels rather than lies. Shakti's legs therefore go over Shiva's thighs. Sir Richard Burton, co-translator of the *Ananga Ranga*, added a footnote that squatting 'upon both feet, somewhat like a bird' was a position 'impossible to Europeans'. Given that he had been a considerable athlete, that's quite surprising because squatting is, in fact, extremely easy, especially with a little help from the hands. Shakti's buttocks, of course, need to be raised up on a pillow or two. One advantage of squatting is that a greater variety of movements is possible. Another is that Shiva's buttocks, scrotum and anal area become easily available to Shakti's caresses. When you, Shiva, get tired you can vary things by squatting on one leg with the other out behind (in a lunging position) or seamlessly switch to a kneeling position.

SAMAPADA-UTTANA-BANDHA

As for *veshtita asana*, Shakti lies on her back with a pillow under her buttocks but this time she places her open legs on Shiva's shoulders.

VYOMAPADA-UTTANA-BANDHA

This is a more extreme development of the previous position. Shakti places her hands around the backs of her knees, or even around her feet, and pulls her legs right back to her head (or as close as she can manage). By doing so, she presents Shiva with a highly erotic view and opens herself for really deep penetration.

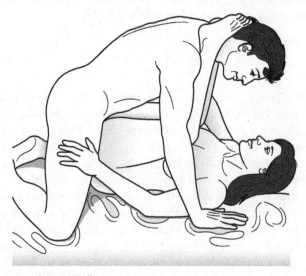

Figure 10.6 Vyomapada-uttana-bandha.

SPHUTMA-UTTANA-BANDHA

This is another progression from *samapada-uttana-bandha*. Shiva places both of Shakti's legs together and holds them straight up. This creates a quite different sensation for both, since the vagina is now constricted. You, Shiva, can caress Shakti's calves against the side of your face or, lowering her legs a little, you can suck her toes.

All positions in which Shakti lies on her back are known as *uttana-bandha*. You can create numerous variations of your own by adding more cushions, by Shakti pulling her legs further and further back, by her raising just one leg, and so on.

One equal position

There are not many genuinely 'equal' ways of making love but this is certainly one. *Both* of you, Shiva and Shakti, get on hands and knees and reverse up to one another. Shiva then swings his *lingam* right around between his legs as far as it will go and inserts it into the *yoni*. It needs a *lingam* of at least average size and it works best with a taller man and a shorter woman, otherwise it's hard to get things aligned. Shaktis are used to adopting this position for rear-entry sex but for Shivas it will be novel. Shiva experiences the sort of 'open' sensation that women get while Shakti feels intense pressure on her G-spot. You can both reach between your legs to stimulate one another and yourselves or you can reach around behind and feel one another that way.

Warning: A word of warning to Shiva – it's better not to ejaculate in this position as the *lingam* is somewhat constricted.

More standing positions

We've already taken a look at *dhenuka-vyanta-bandha* (see p. 223) in which Shakti stands, bends forwards, and supports herself on anything convenient. Generally, standing positions aren't very Tantric because they can't be held for long. But they can be an exciting part of a sequence of *asanas* and are especially useful out-of-doors.

HARI-VIKRAMA-UTTHITA-BANDHA

Shakti raises one leg and curls it around Shiva's hip (or even higher if she's a dancer or contortionist). This swings the *yoni* sufficiently forward for Shiva to enter with his *lingam*.

KIRTI-UTTHITA-BANDHA

Shakti places her hands on Shiva's shoulders and springs up, putting her legs around his waist. Shiva, placing his hands under her buttocks, manoeuvres her onto his *lingam*. If there's a convenient wall or tree he can lean back against it for support, in which case Shakti can put her feet against it to move herself backwards and forwards.

Adhorata positions

Given that the *yoni* and the anus are close together, it seems logical that any position that works for the former should also work for *adhorata*. But, in fact, there are some special considerations, due to the fact that, although the rectum and vagina run more or less parallel, the anus itself is at an angle. Even more important, although it's easy for the *lingam* to find its way into an unseen *yoni*, it's extremely difficult to penetrate the anal sphincters if you can't see what you're doing. That's why, in the previous chapter, I suggested you start with the lordosis position. (Remember that copious amounts of artificial lubricant are absolutely essential.)

LORDOSIS (ANAL VERSION)

This is the same posture as for vaginal sex described above. In fact, having given Shakti a vaginal orgasm in this position, it's a seamless move for Shiva to switch to anal penetration. To prepare

Shakti, tantalize her anal area with a lubricated finger ('anal hand', remember!) while *lingam* and *yoni* are united, then slip the finger inside. After a while it may be helpful to add a second finger, and even a third. (For full details of anal foreplay see the previous chapter.) Once the sphincter is relaxed, slowly withdraw the finger(s), use plenty of lubricant on the *lingam* and insert as gently as possible.

VYOMAPADA-UTTANA-BANDHA *(ANAL VERSION)*

On her back, with a pillow under her buttocks, Shakti places her hands around the backs of her knees, or even around her feet, and pulls her legs right back to her head (or as close as she can manage). By doing so, she presents Shiva with clear access to her anus.

TIRYAKASANA *(ANAL VERSION)*

In this variation on the sideways theme, Shakti lies with her buttocks right on the edge of the bed, her legs a little bent. Shiva stands or kneels on the floor, raises Shakti's upper leg a little, and inserts himself. (A pillow or two may be necessary to get things to line up.)

PURUSHAYITA-BHRAMARA-BANDHA *(ANAL VERSION)*

This is the most Tantric of the anal positions because it puts the woman on top. But it's also the most difficult because neither Shakti/Kali nor Shiva can see what's going on. Everything has to be done by feel. You, Shakti/Kali, order your man to lie flat on his back, straddle him and squat down on your feet. Shiva will need to hold his *lingam* steady in his hand while you manoeuvre. When you feel the head of the *lingam* on your anus, gently lower yourself by degrees. Shiva can give support by taking a buttock in each hand. You, Shakti/Kali, can increase your pleasure by playing with your *yonimani* and breasts.

Rather than merely relax the sphincter, it may help to actually bear down with your 'anal muscles' which should cause the anus to open a little.

10 THINGS TO REMEMBER

1 *The most Tantric positions are the ones in which the woman – the goddess – is in charge.*

2 *The 'secret language' requires Shakti to develop her muscles such that she can stroke the* lingam *inside her* yoni.

3 *Different positions offer different possibilities for breath control, the intoning of mantras, the meeting of eyes, energy circulation and altered states of consciousness.*

4 *Static goddess-on-top positions are excellent for long, meditative sessions.*

5 *There are also goddess-on-top positions in which Shakti can be very active, taking her pleasure exactly as she wishes.*

6 *When Shakti is active on top she needs considerable skill to bring her partner to the edge of ejaculation again and again; good communication is vital.*

7 *Older men may find it difficult to sustain goddess-on-top positions since gravity is opposing the blood supply to the* lingam.

8 *When Shiva is in control, he can more easily get very close to the PNR.*

9 *In Tantric sex, whenever appropriate, men squat rather than kneel or lie.*

10 Adhorata *is theoretically possible in most of the positions used for vaginal sex but in practice it helps enormously for Shiva to be able to see what he's doing.*

HOW TANTRIC ARE YOU NOW?

☐ (Women only) Have you developed the ability to 'speak' the secret language?

☐ (Men only) Can you reply to the 'secret language' so that Shakti can really get the message?

☐ Have you stared unblinking into one another's eyes for two minutes during intercourse?

☐ Have you tried a goddess-on-top position in which neither of you moved for several minutes?

☐ Have you tried a goddess-on-top position in which Shakti alone did the moving?

☐ (Women only) Have you taken complete charge of a Tantric sex session, telling your man exactly what you want him to do?

☐ Have you been able to lie still in a position such as the X and move energy?

☐ Have you tried a rear-entry position?

☐ Have you tried a sideways position?

☐ Have you tried a standing position?

☐ Have you tried at least two different positions for *adhorata*?

☐ (Men only) Have you tried squatting rather than kneeling or lying?

If you answered 'yes' to between eight and ten questions you're obviously very open to Tantric sex ideas and have worked hard on acquiring the skills.

If you answered 'yes' to between five and seven questions you're on your way but you have quite a bit of experimenting and practising to do.

If you couldn't answer 'yes' to more than four questions, maybe you're thinking there's nothing wrong with the good old missionary. In that case, read the chapter again and at least try *some* new positions. Remember that Tantric sex is partly about opening your mind to new ideas.

11

The seven stages of bliss

In this chapter you will learn:
- *what bliss is*
- *how to create a complete Tantric sex session*
- *how you can reach the highest levels of bliss.*

> *There is but one thing which all seek – happiness – though it be of differing kinds and sought in different ways. All forms, whether sensual, intellectual, or spiritual, are from the Brahman, who is Itself the Source and Essence of all Bliss, and Bliss itself... and thus it is said that man can never be truly happy until he seeks shelter with Brahman, which is Itself the great Bliss.*
>
> Arthur Avalon (Sir John Woodroffe), introduction to the *Mahanirvana Tantra*

So now we're going to pull together everything you've been practising for the greatest evening (or afternoon or morning) of *ananda* you've had so far. As I've been stressing throughout the book, *ananda* is the whole point of Tantric sex. It's not the same thing as happiness and it's not the same thing as the physical excitement a woman feels as she orgasms or a man feels as he ejaculates. *Ananda* is an intensely beautiful altered state of consciousness, brought about by Tantric sex, although separate from the sexual feelings.

But what actually is it? First of all I'll give you the Tantric outlook. Then I'll give you an alternative, scientific Western outlook.

The early Tantrikas had a very specific view of *ananda*. 'Ananda,' wrote Abhinavagupta, the Tantric sage, 'is the supreme Brahman'. Some Tantrikas sought it entirely through meditation, some through mantras, and some through sex. We're obviously interested in pursuing it through sex which, as the thirteenth century guru Jayaratha put it, brings not only 'pleasure in a worldly sense,' but also 'absorption into the very nature of undivided supreme consciousness.'

In other words, traditional Tantrikas believe that when you experience *ananda* you experience the Divine Consciousness, God, or whatever term you prefer. They believe that when Brahman created the universe 'he' created it out of 'himself'. After all, there wasn't anything else. So Tantrikas believe the universe is the body of Brahman. They believe their own bodies are microcosms of the universe. They believe they're part of Brahman. They believe they *are* Brahman and that, through Tantric sex, they experience that truth directly. That's the whole significance of the mantra *So Hum*, meaning 'I am Brahman' in the same sense that a single cell of your body, complete with all your DNA, is you. They believe their bliss is just a foretaste of the bliss that awaits them when they achieve *moksha*, or liberation from the cycle of death and rebirth.

Now here's the scientific view. When you make love the Tantric way for, let's say three hours, you flood your brain with a powerful cocktail of pleasure-giving chemicals. Let's take a closer look at the most important ones:

▶ **Dopamine**, *the primary bliss chemical, gets into the frontal lobe of the brain during* nyasa, *during orgasm and, crucially, in the moment before orgasm, which is why 'surfing' the pre-orgasmic millisecond produces such a rapture (but in men more than women). Dopamine is so potent that rats, wired up to be able to stimulate the 'pleasure centres' of their own brains, will continue doing so until, never stopping to eat or drink, they, as it were, die of ecstasy.*
▶ **PEA**, *an amphetamine-like substance that makes you feel like you're walking on air, builds up throughout* nyasa *and peaks at orgasm. The longer the* nyasa, *the more of this you'll have, and the more you'll maintain (or get back) those euphoric*

feelings from the early days of your love affair. PEA combined with dopamine and the stress-reducing noradrenaline makes an even more potent combination. (Incidentally, you can increase your noradrenaline level by ten times with just eight minutes of vigorous exercise.)

▶ **Oxytocin** *is the sensitizing hormone because it makes your skin more responsive, the romantic hormone because it makes you feel bonded with your partner, and the orgasmic hormone because it powers the contractions. Again, it's built up during* nyasa, *simply by touching and stroking and kissing. That makes it self-reinforcing. The longer you do it, the better it feels. A large dose can also make you 'spaced-out'.*

▶ **Serotonin** *is a complicated neurotransmitter. It has a role to play in happiness and in mystical feelings, but although it goes up in men during sex, it can go* down *when men ejaculate.*

Clearly, then, the longer you have sex, the more these chemicals build up. So is Tantric sex a 'drug trip'? Yes it is. There's no denying it.

But could Tantric sex be more than that? Is it the case that the 'drugs' damage our powers of perception and reasoning, causing us to hallucinate? Or is it the case that the 'drugs' *facilitate* our powers of perception and reasoning, allowing us to comprehend things which otherwise would be beyond us? Is it the case that the particular altered state of consciousness depends on the psychological techniques used before and during sex? Or do those techniques just help us to see more clearly? In other words, do we dissolve into our partners because we expect to? Do we experience the Divine Consciousness because we expect to? Or is there something genuine going on?

You decide.

An evening of Tantric sex

According to Abhinavagupta, there are actually seven levels of *ananda*. The first level, ***nijananda***, was the bliss experienced by Brahman before the creation of the visible universe. So that's not really available to humans. You would therefore start at the second level, *nirananda*, literally 'non-bliss'.

Let's spy, then, on a Tantric couple and see how they progress from *nirananda* to *jagadananda*, the seventh and ultimate level. Although you've now, presumably, read all about the various practices, some of the things they do may still seem a little weird and you certainly don't have to copy them exactly. They're just to inspire you and demonstrate how all the elements you've learned fit together into a Tantric sex session. But, as time goes on, you'll probably feel more and more comfortable with the Tantric rituals and increasingly include them in your lovemaking.

7.30 a.m.
Shiva and Shakti awake. They've been sleeping naked side-by-side, so it's very easy to reach out to one another and press skin against skin. Soon *yoni* and *lingam* are briefly united and as the lovers look into each other's eyes so they make an assignation for the evening.

Insight

You've learned how, in traditional Tantra, the visible universe is nothing more than a web of vibrations created by the lovemaking of the gods. If they ever stop making those vibrations then the universe will implode. And that's a very good allegory for any romantic relationship. You've got to keep making those vibrations. Why not unite *lingam* and *yoni* for a minute or two every day, or even twice a day? Not every lovemaking has to be a full Tantric ritual. Starting the day like this not only means starting the day very happily, it reinforces your whole Tantric way of being.

6.00 p.m.
Shiva and Shakti assemble the accessories they're going to need:

▶ *wine*
▶ *a 'Tantric' goblet that's never used on any other occasion*
▶ *some 'Tantric' appetizers on a 'Tantric' plate*
▶ *candles*
▶ *incense*

- *jewellery*
- *a crop-top for Shakti, an embroidered waistcoat for Shiva*
- *body oil or cream for nyasa*
- *a CD of romantic Eastern music.*

Insight

Tantric sex is always a very special occasion. The right accessories underline that and focus your minds on what you're hoping to achieve. But, in addition, they extend the range of sensual inputs and, therefore, increase the likelihood of reaching that ultimate level of bliss. Pay attention to your choice of music – the right kind can help extend the altered state of consciousness once sex is over.

6.30 p.m.
The Tantric couple make a little time to meditate on what they're going to be doing and why. Shiva goes to his laptop and meditates on a *yantra* (Chapter 4) he made himself from a digital image of his partner's *yoni*. Shakti prefers to meditate in the traditional way, sitting in the half lotus.

Insight

This is a key moment in Tantric sex. You need to focus on the kind of spiritual experience you would like to have during the *maithuna* that follows. Additionally, if there's something you particularly want to achieve, or if you're anxious about an issue, then this is the opportunity to enlist the help of your unconscious mind. Shiva is concerned about losing control so, fixing his gaze on his *yantra*, he visualizes his *lingam* sliding in and out endlessly until he and Shakti have both reached a state of bliss. He could also have tried putting himself into a trance (see Chapter 8). Meanwhile, Shakti is eager to experience such a sense of oneness with her partner that she'll no longer know where her body ends and where her partner's body begins. She meditates on her body as mostly empty space, merging into the space that is her partner. (When you meditate like this, make sure you give yourselves enough time afterwards to shake off any meditative sleepiness.)

7.00 p.m.

The moment has come for Shiva and Shakti to come together to share food and drink and to challenge themselves by breaking a taboo (Chapter 3). Shakti pours a little red wine into the goblet, licks a finger in a tantalizing way, and uses it to stir the wine. Shiva licks his finger and does the same. They take turns to sip the wine, kissing it into one another's mouths. Likewise with the food. Shakti takes a morsel into her mouth, bites a piece off, swallows it, and kisses what's left into her partner's mouth. Shiva bites it again, returning a quarter. What taboo will they break? Shiva wants to watch a few minutes of an erotic film. He's eager to see Shakti's reaction to a scene in which two women make love and one of them ejaculates a stream of fluid. Shakti has never done that yet and he wants to talk about how it might be possible. But Shakti is already recounting a fantasy in which, out clothes shopping with a girlfriend, they share a changing room...

Level of bliss: *Parananda*, the third, or the bliss that's initiated by external things.

Insight

When you swallow something from your partner's body, your partner literally becomes a part of you. Reflect on the incredible significance of that for a moment. The intention behind Tantric sex is not so much to unite male and female as to *reunite* because, in the beginning, was the *Ardhanari*, the androgen, whose left side was female and whose right side was male, and who was split in half. The breaking of taboos, too, is a way of opening your mind to new ideas as well as of sharing your deepest and most private thoughts and feelings. Anything you can do to eliminate that sense of separation from your 'other half' will help destroy loneliness. And, of course, the sharing of food and wine, and the joint breaking of taboos, create a delicious sexy frisson and the stirrings of *rasa* in our Tantric couple.

7.30 p.m.
Shiva and Shakti undress to shower together. Shakti's pubic hair is covering the lips of her *yoni*, but Shiva wants to be able to see clearly. He trims her locks with her electric razor. When he's finished she steps under the hot jet and washes the cut hairs away. Shiva joins her and they soap one another, enjoying the sensation of their hands gliding over each other's wet, slippery bodies.

7.45 p.m.
Shiva puts on some music. Shakti lights the candles and the incense so the room seems to flicker in a warm, aromatic glow. Shiva puts on his waistcoat and some silver bracelets. Shakti puts on the crop-top, a necklace, a chain around her waist, and a strand of tinkling bells around her left ankle.

It's vital to create the right atmosphere. Choose the music carefully. It should be both sensual and mystical, helping to suck you into an altered state of consciousness. Likewise the candles, the incense and the accessories, which should be reserved for Tantric sex sessions only. (In the daytime it will help to draw the curtains so you can enjoy the candlelight.)

7.55 p.m.
Shakti sits up on the bed, leaning back against cushions, displaying her newly-shaved *yoni*. Shiva, bowing down before her, takes her left foot, places it on his head and announces, 'This is the foot of my goddess, *OM*.' He intones the mantra in the proper way, 'Aah-oh-ong', and feels the vibrations spreading down his chest. He puts her big toe in his mouth and sucks it. He takes a little massage cream and rubs it into her foot...

Insight

This is the beginning of *nyasa*, as described in Chapter 5. It's a combination of sexual foreplay and spiritual rite, identifying each partner with the divine. Really try to feel every cell with your fingertips because it's in so doing that you maximize the production of oxytocin which, later on, will fire the orgasmic contractions. And even if you have no religious or spiritual beliefs at all you should still say something to express your appreciation for your partner, as you stimulate different parts of the body. Shakti is not in the least inhibited about displaying her *yoni* (nor is Shiva inhibited about displaying his *lingam*). Shakti knows that, in the words of the *Candamaharosana Tantra*, her 'three-petalled lotus' (the two inner labia and the hood of the clitoris) is a 'Buddha paradise' that 'bestows bliss'.

8.10 p.m.

Shiva places a cushion under Shakti's buttocks and lying between her open thighs begins *auparishtaka* (Chapter 6). At first he tantalizes her by intoning a mantra while pressing his lips against her *yoni*. Next, he runs the very tip of his tongue up and down the whole length of it. Gently pushing her thighs to tip her a little backwards, he includes her anal area. Deep inside her, in the region of the *Muladhara* chakra, *Kundalini* stirs. Placing his left hand on her pubic mound he presses it upwards so as to retract the hood of her *yonimani* and reveal the tiny red jewel itself. Flicking his tongue over it faster and faster he causes *Kundalini* to rise up and pierce *Swadisthana*, the second chakra, giving Shakti her first orgasm and flooding her *yoni* with juice. The Tantric couple adjust their positions and Shakti now lies between Shiva's thighs and takes his *lingam* into her mouth. While she plays her wet tongue over his glans she pours lubricant into her hand and fondles his scrotum and anal area. In Shiva, too, *Kundalini* stirs and the *Muladhara* chakra opens.

Insight

As we saw in Chapter 2, *Kundalini* is sexual energy, envisaged as a serpent goddess lying asleep at the base of the spine. Stimulating the anal area simultaneously with the genitals is the fast route to arousing 'her'.

8.30 p.m.

Shiva and Shakti are now united in the position known as *yab yum*. Shiva sits upright on the bed with his legs crossed while

Shakti sits on his lap, *lingam* in *yoni*, her legs crossed behind him. They gaze deeply into one another's eyes. They are locked together at every point – tongues, breasts, arms, genitals. Their breathing is synchronized. Together they breathe in and out, deeply and rapidly without pauses, for five minutes, willing the energy to circulate right through them. Then, clasping one another's wrists, they lean backwards until their heads touch the bed and her heels press hard into his sacrum. This is the static variation of the position known as *mula bandha*, and they hold it for 15 minutes, their legs tingling and their minds turned inwards on a voyage of discovery. As Shiva feels a tiny quantity of sexual fluid seep out of his *lingam* he knows that his *Swadisthana* chakra, too, has opened.

Level of bliss: **Brahmananda**, the fourth, or the bliss that comes from the revelation of the true self.

Insight

Lying still in *mula bandha*, Shiva and Shakti become aware, as Abhinavagupta put it, of their 'own nature' that is, their inner selves. And what is that? For Tantrikas, it's Brahman. One perspective, given by Alice Bunker Stockham (see Chapter 7), is that the 'quiet union of the sexual organs' leads to 'the knowledge of the living, spiritual truth that man has no separate existence from God.' If you have neither religious nor spiritual beliefs, you can simply try to turn off your thoughts, 'look' inwards and see what happens.

9.00 p.m.
Shiva and Shakti switch to *samapada-uttana-bandha* (Shakti on her back with her legs on Shiva's shoulders). Slowly, Shiva thrusts, sometimes keeping just inside the entrance to Shakti's *yoni*, pressing the head of his *lingam* against her G-spot, sometimes sliding all the way in to her cervix. Shiva feels himself become more and more excited. With a few more thrusts he takes himself right to the razor's edge of ejaculation and it's there he intends to stay, surfing on a wave of pleasure. They stare intently into one another's eyes, moving by millimetres, watching for the first sign of orgasm. Shakti lets out a little moan and Shiva feels her starting

to come. He arches his back in the locking position as a chemical charge shoots into his brain and his eyes roll up. But the locking position won't be enough and he thrusts his tongue out and down and exhales violently several times. Close. Very close. And so they go on. And with each orgasm the chemicals build up until their brains are awash with dopamine. Now they roll into *vinaka-tiryak-bandha* (sideways), and Shiva bends his leg and slides it up over Shakti's hip, thus exposing his anal area to her fingers. He reaches for the bottle of lubricant, applies some to himself, then pours some more onto his own fingers and reaches around under Shakti's buttocks. As she slides a forefinger into Shiva's anal canal she feels Shiva do the same to her. *Kundalini* rises to a whole new level, piercing the *Manipura* chakra at the solar plexus.

Level of bliss: *Mahananda*, the fifth, the bliss that's initiated by being totally absorbed in one another. Nothing else exists but the two of them.

Insight

For a woman, what does it feel like to experience an orgasm that is at once both physical and spiritual? Perhaps like this:

> *I saw in his hand a long spear of gold, and at the iron's point there seemed to be a little fire. He appeared to me to be thrusting it at times into my heart, and to pierce my very entrails; when he drew it out, he seemed to draw them out also, and to leave me all on fire with a great love of Brahman. The pain was so great, that it made me moan; and yet so surpassing was the sweetness of this excessive pain, that I could not wish to be rid of it...*

In fact, that was a description of her 'raptures' written by St Teresa of Avila (1515–82), except that I've substituted '*Brahman*' for 'God'. Whether or not it was truly a description of an orgasm it certainly reads very much like it. And that, really, is the point. The physical experience of orgasm and the mental experience of an altered state of consciousness can be closely linked.

9.30 p.m.

Without disengaging, the Tantric couple roll over again into the lordosis position. Shiva drips lubricant between Shakti's buttocks and she spreads her legs a little wider, concentrating now on raising *Kundalini* still higher, focusing on her love for Shiva and her desire to manifest that love through her body. She feels Shiva's finger once again penetrate her anus, then two fingers, then three, gently and unhurriedly preparing her for *adhorata*. Soon he slides out of her *yoni* and she feels the head of his *lingam* tantalizing her anal area and then, with a little thrust, he's inside. For two or three minutes, neither of them moves as she adjusts to the new sensations. Then she herself begins thrusting back against him. Shiva slips a finger inside her *yoni* and presses her G-spot as she reaches between her legs to rub her *yonimani*. Shiva lies along her back, taking her hair in his hands, gently biting her neck and ears. He, too, is full of love. The *Anahata* or heart chakra has been pierced. This is the most intimate act they can perform. Shakti has offered herself utterly and completely. In so doing she has achieved her wish that there should be no physical barrier between them. Shakti orgasms again.

Level of bliss: *Cidananda*, the sixth, the bliss that's initiated by total fusion. They are one.

9.45 p.m.

Shiva and Shakti shower again together, share a little food and drink, and return to the bed. Shakti displays her *yoni* once more while Shiva masturbates to erection. He slides into her and gently nudges her backwards into *vyomapada-uttana-banda*, so that her knees are close to her ears. As he begins slow thrusting, so *Kundalini* quickly regains the level of the *Anahata* chakra and they each now concentrate on driving the 'serpent' still higher. Time and again they take one another to the brink – Shakti to the brink of orgasm, Shiva to the brink of ejaculation. They're literally delirious with pleasure, as if they had drunk *soma*, the intoxicant loved by the gods. The *Vishuddhi* chakra, the gateway to transcendence, has opened. They're no longer in the everyday world. The longing to experience simultaneous orgasm becomes intense. Shiva increases his thrusting. He's been in a state of continuous arousal for three hours and his *lingam* has been receiving direct stimulation for some 100 minutes. The degree of vasocongestion (blood in the genital area) has become enormous. His prostate is bursting with fluid. Shiva lets out a scream as his *lingam* begins pumping. Swept along by the energy, Shakti, too, begins her final orgasm. In both of them the *Ajna* chakra opens. The orgasm goes on and on. They are in a void. Their bodies no longer exist. The bed, the bedroom, the house...none of it exists. Time no longer exists. The *Sahasrara* has opened. They have achieved *samadhi*.

Level of bliss: *Jagadananda*, the seventh, the bliss of cosmic oneness.

10.00 p.m.
Shiva and Shakti lie unmoving for a long while, overcome by the *rasa*-juice that seems to have flooded their brains. They are unaware of their surroundings. Their bodies are as if dead to them, heavy and burdensome. They are almost pure mind, glowing and radiant. Minutes pass. Five, ten... Eventually, they struggle to move, see one another once more, resume the *yab yum* posture (now without the *lingam* in the *yoni*), feed one another little treats and kiss wine into one another's mouths.

Insight

On this occasion, Shiva eventually ejaculated, as he had planned all along. He feels no sense of let-down but only bliss because he's left what for him is the correct interval since his last ejaculation. The next time he has sex (maybe tomorrow) he won't ejaculate. Nor the time after that. Nor maybe the time after that. Every Shiva has to know his own body and ejaculate at the intervals that will ensure bliss, without risking any sense of let-down or of the sexual hangover (Chapter 7). If this had been a non-ejaculatory Tantric session, Shiva would still have been able to achieve *jagadananda* and *samadhi* through the cumulative effect of multiple orgasms. Of course, in reality, the attainment of the ultimate state is rare. The session described above is an ideal. But if you follow all the advice in this book you should normally be able to achieve *mahananda* and, quite often, *cidananda*.

DOES TANTRIC SEX REALLY HAVE TO
BE THIS LONG?

You probably have more time for sex than you think. It's a question of prioritizing it. But, no, Tantric sex doesn't have to last three hours. It's simply a question of how long it takes to build that radically altered state of consciousness. It's unlikely to be less than one hour. On the other hand, if you have sex frequently, say every day, with a Tantric outlook, and if you maintain the sexual buzz in your relationship, then your whole life becomes a Tantric sex session. When that happens, a 'quickie' is no longer a 'quickie' but one element of a Tantric sex session that never ends. So along with 'slowies' you can still have 'quickies' (probably without ejaculation). In fact, you should.

Some personal experiences of bliss

The Tantric states of bliss are difficult to convey in words but here some men and women from my focus groups have a go:

> *Every time I'm on the verge of ejaculating I get this tremendous hit of chemicals in the brain. Once I've done that about six times in a row I feel I must have died and gone to Paradise.*

> *I begin with clitoral orgasms and then go on to vaginal. With each one there's more and more a change of consciousness. Eventually I'm not aware of anything going on around me but seem to be inside a vast inner space.*

> *On one occasion the blissful state went on for several hours. It was almost frightening at first because it seemed I'd*

literally lost touch with reality. Then I realized that, on the contrary, I was only just starting to perceive reality.

Some of the bliss for me is in making my partner so excited. He has multiple orgasms and gets completely spaced out and that makes me spaced out too.

I feel as if I'm on the verge of solving the mystery of the universe, but I never quite manage it. Which is good, because it means I have to keep on trying.

Arousal is the ultimate in Tantric sex as far as I'm concerned. I would give up orgasms rather than this feeling I get.

I feel that my ordinary cares and anxieties are of no significance; I feel beyond harm.

During Tantric sex there's this tremendous excitement but afterwards it becomes a very quiet sort of happiness, as if I know a special secret.

When we do the meeting of eyes it's like I'm something separate from my body looking out from inside, and my partner is something separate from his body, and then we really make contact in a way that never happens otherwise.

I had 'normal' sex for thirty years, thinking ejaculation was the whole point. Now I don't care if I never ejaculate again. All I want is for those sort of Tantric sensations to keep on and on and on.

I feel embarrassed about saying this, but I feel a love for the whole universe and, what sounds even more weird, I feel the universe loves me. I don't feel in the universe, I feel part of the universe.

Final word

A Tantrika is more than someone who practices Tantric sex from time to time. The blissful state of consciousness I experience after Tantric sex may only last from a few minutes up to half an hour (and occasionally several hours), but Tantric sex is like throwing the proverbial stone into the proverbial pond. The vibrations spread out and out. After I'd had my first experience of *ananda*, my whole view of life changed a little. Now that I've had many experiences of *ananda* it has changed a lot. I'm sure the same will happen to you.

Ananda!

10 THINGS TO REMEMBER

1 *According to Abhinavagupta there were seven levels of bliss.*

2 *Try to unite* lingam *and* yoni *every day – it helps maintain the Tantric way of being and is very good for a relationship.*

3 *Tantric sex sessions aren't spontaneous but need planning.*

4 *Take pleasure in assembling your food, drink and accessories – and do it in good time.*

5 *Prepare yourselves for Tantric sex through meditation and then by intimately sharing wine and food and by breaking a taboo.*

6 *It's vital to create the right mystical ambience with music, candles, incense and suitable accessories.*

7 *Acknowledge your partner as a god/goddess.*

8 *Allow plenty of time for a full Tantric sex session – even as much as three hours.*

9 *The altered state of consciousness you experience in Tantric sex depends on the psychological techniques used before and during sex.*

10 *Mystical experiences of Tantric bliss are difficult to convey in words.*

HOW TANTRIC ARE YOU NOW?

- [ ] Have you been able to generate *parananda*, the bliss that comes from external things such as sharing food, wine and confidences?
- [ ] Have you been able to generate *brahmananda*, the bliss that comes from insight into your inner self?
- [ ] Have you been able to generate *mahananda*, the bliss that comes from intense involvement with your partner?
- [ ] Have you been able to generate *cidananda*, the bliss that comes from total fusion?
- [ ] Have you been able to generate *jagadananda*, the bliss that comes from the realization of oneness with the cosmos?

Whatever level you've reached so far the advice is the same. Keep on learning about Tantric sex and keep on doing it. The more often you have Tantric sex the more your life will be full of bliss.

Glossary

Abhinavagupta: Tantric sage (c. 960–c.1020 CE) who wrote the *Tantraloka*.

abhiseka: Tantric empowerment ritual.

ahimsa: Hindu doctrine of non-violence.

Ajna: the sixth **chakra** situated between and slightly above the eyebrows.

Anahata: the fourth **chakra** situated near the heart.

ananda: bliss – the aim of Tantric sex.

apana: one of the forms of energy in the **subtle body**, filling the area around the anus.

asana: posture.

Atharva Veda: the fourth *Veda*, dealing with magic and medicine.

atman: the self, soul or spirit.

bandha: a muscular lock or contraction, to control the flow of *prana*; can be used to prolong sex.

Bhagavadgita: a mystical poem, forming part of the *Mahabharata*.

Bhairava: effectively the ultimate reality; **Bhairava** is surrounded by bhairavas as his circle of attendants (see **Shiva**).

bhakti: the path of **Yoga** that seeks enlightenment through devotion.

bhoga: Sanskrit word which can mean both 'food' and 'sexual pleasure', leading to ambiguity in translations.

bija **mantra**: a seed **mantra** or Sanskrit letter denoting a deity.

bindu: the creative male energy whose physical manifestation is semen.

bodhicitta: a state of enlightenment which can be related to semen.

bodhisattva: in Buddhism someone who, although able to attain the state of **nirvana**, remains on Earth to help others.

brahma: in Hinduism the ultimate and impersonal divine reality of the universe.

Brahman: another word for *brahma*; also a member of the highest priestly caste (alternative spelling – Brahmin).

brahmananda: the bliss that comes from the revelation of your true self.

brahmarendra: the 'cavity of Brahman', an area of the brain believed to be responsible for mystical experiences.

Buddha: founder of Buddhism c.500 BCE.

cakrapuja: 'circle worship' – Tantric sex performed as a group.

chakra: a meeting point between mind and body; an energy centre in the **subtle body** (alternative spelling – cakra).

cidananda: the bliss that's initiated by total fusion with your partner.

cosmogram: a diagram representing the structure of the universe.

Dakini: semi-divine beings who eat raw flesh.

dasa: name given by the invading Aryans to the indigenous tribes of India; in the *Rig Veda*, the forces of Evil.

deva: divine male figure.

devi: divine female figure.

dharana: concentration.

dhyana: meditation.

diksa: Tantric initiation ritual.

dravyam: fluid (sexual fluid).

Durga: one of the names for the Great Goddess.

duti: one of several names for the female partner in Tantric rites.

female ejaculation: expulsion of liquid from the urethra by women during sex, either from the Skene's glands (female prostate) or from the bladder, or both.

Gopi: any one of the cowgirls with whom **Krishna** had sex.

G-spot: named after the German researcher Ernst Gräfenberg, it's the small, slightly rough area just inside the entrance of the vagina on the front wall – on the other side of the wall lies the female prostate.

guna: one of the three qualities (*sattva*, *rajas* and *tamas*) that make up the physical universe.

guru: religious teacher and spiritual guide; considered essential for a full understanding of **Tantra**.

Ham Sa: a mantra meaning 'I am He (Brahman).' See also *So Hum*. In meditation pronounce 'Hum' on the exhalation and 'So' on the inhalation.

I Ching: an ancient book of Chinese oracles, also known as *The Book Of Changes*.

ida: one of the major *nadis*, conveying cooling, intuitive, feminine energy up the left side of the spine and out through the left nostril.

Indra: king of the Vedic gods.

jagadananda: the bliss of cosmic oneness.

jaina: a religion, founded c.500 BCE by Mahavira, in which the monks strive not to harm any living creature (also known as **Jainism**).

japa: repetition of a **mantra** to fix it in the subconscious.

Jayaratha: Tantric **guru** (c.1225–c.1275 CE) who wrote a commentary to the *Tantraloka*.

jiva: a human being, that is, the physical embodiment of the *atma*; an individual soul.

jivanmukti: bodily immortality.

kalacakra: in Tantric Buddhism a system of *mandalas* and meditations.

Kali: the 'Terrible Goddess'.

kama: love.

kanda: 'bulb'; the sex organ.

karma: the sum total of good and bad deeds performed by an individual during various incarnations and which will have an impact on the next incarnation.

kaula: the hard core of sexual practices within **Tantra**.

khecara: flight (one of the goals of the early Tantrikas).

Krishna: a god and an alternative incarnation of **Vishnu** (alternative spelling – Krisna).

kriya: a purification practice.

kula: an extensive family or clan of Tantrikas.

kuladravyam: the 'clan fluid', that is, the divine essence embodied in the vaginal fluid; also known as *yonitattva* (vulval essence) or simply *dravyam* (fluid).

Kundalini: energy, untapped in most people, that lies coiled at the base of the spine and which can be awoken by Tantric sex (also *Candalini*).

Kundalini **gland**: a knot of blood vessels between the rectum and the base of the spine, believed by Tantrikas to be the source of the euphoric energy that is released during sex (alternative names – coccygeal body or Luschka's body).

laya **yoga**: system of **yoga** that transmutes lower forms of energy into higher forms.

left-hand path: style of **Tantra** in which men and women who may not be committed to one another have sex for the achievement of *ananda*.

lila: erotic play.

lingam: penis.

mahabrahmanda: the cosmos; *mahabrahmanda* contains myriad *brihatbrahmanda* or microcosms; every person is a microcosm of the cosmos.

mahananda: the bliss initiated by becoming totally intent on one another.

maharaga: the highest and most passionate form of energy; an inner state in which the ultimate reality can be experienced.

mahavidya: the energy of the Great Goddess in female form.

maithuna: sexual union.

mandala: a circular diagram used for concentrating energy.

mani: penis; in Tantric Buddhism, an insight. Literally, jewel.

Manipura: the third **chakra**, at the solar plexus.

mantra: a sound, word or phrase used to create special vibrations.

maya: the covering that conceals the true nature of the universe.

melaka or melana or melapa: mingling (of men and women i.e. sex).

merudanda: the spinal tube in the **subtle body**, identified with Meru, the mythical mountain at the centre of the universe, from which all water flows.

million dollar point: modern name for the point between the anus and scrotum where pressure can be applied to the prostate (I don't recommend this – see Chapter 8).

moksha: liberation from the cycle of death and rebirth.

mudra: a special gesture that can concentrate energy; can also mean the vulva.

mukham: mouth.

mukti: rebirth.

mula: 'root'; the sex organ.

Muladhara: the lowest or root **chakra** situated near to the anus.

multiple orgasms: the bursts of pleasure-giving chemicals in the brain that accompany the contractions that precede ejaculation.

nadi: channel in the **subtle body** through which energies flow.

nijananda: the bliss enjoyed by **Brahman** before creating the universe.

nirananda: non-bliss.

nirvana: in Buddhism, the ultimate state of release.

nyasa: a ritual touching of various parts of a partner's body, identifying them with those of a deity.

OM: the original and most powerful of all **mantras**.

padma: the lotus; an alternative name for a **chakra**; vulva/penis (since the flower expands and contracts).

Padmini: lotus woman (a beautiful woman).

pancatattva: the 'left-handed' Tantric rite in which couples, seated in a circle around their **guru**, have ritualistic sex, possibly with partners other than their spouses.

parananda: the bliss that's initiated by external pleasures.

paravritti: utilizing the energies of the **subtle body** that would otherwise be wasted.

Parvati: the Goddess in the form of the wife of **Shiva**.

pashu/pasu: follower at the lowest level and considered a 'brute'.

PC muscle: the **pubococcygeus muscle**.

pingala: one of the major *nadis*, conveying hot, rational, male energy up the right side of the spine and out through the right nostril.

pon: gold (i.e. menstrual blood – compare with *velli*).

prakriti: the physical universe; nature.

prana: the energy of the **subtle body**.

pranayama: regulation of breathing; can be used to control ejaculation.

pubococcygeus muscle: in popular use the umbrella name for the group of muscles that, in both men and women, surround and flex the genitals.

puja: the rituals of worship.

pujari: someone who performs *puja*.

purana: collection of Sanskrit myths.

purusha: spirit.

raga: passion. See *maharaga*.

rahasyacarya: 'secret ceremony'; another name for *cakrapuja*.

rajapana: drinking vaginal fluids.

rajas: the *guna* (quality) of activity, passion and change; menstrual blood.

rasa: 'juice-joy'; the ultimate state reached in Tantric sex.

rasa-juice: the nectar that floods down over the brain at the climax to Tantric sex.

right-hand path: style of **Tantra** in which only committed couples have sex for the achievement of *ananda*; some seek *ananda* entirely by non-sexual means such as meditation and **mantras**.

Rig Veda: the earliest of the *Vedas*, dating from around 1200 BCE.

rishis: seers.

sadhaka/sadhika: man/woman who observes the rituals and beliefs of **Tantra**.

sadhana: all the rituals performed by a *sadhaka*.

Sahasrara: the thousand-petalled lotus in the **subtle body** at the crown of the head; considered by some as the seventh and highest **chakra**.

samadhi: 'with God.' A state of superconsciousness following union of the individual consciousness with the universal consciousness.

sattva: the *guna* (quality) of purity.

Shakti: the Great Goddess (alternative spelling – Sakti); the divine energy in female form.

shishya: pupil of a **guru**.

Shiva: the most important male god in Hinduism (alternative spelling – Siva); the ultimate reality.

siddha: perfected being.

siddhis: psychic powers or 'sixth sense'.

So Hum: see *Ham Sa*.

subtle body: a parallel invisible body.

susumna: the central major *nadi*, inside the spine according to some systems, parallel with the spine according to others.

sutra: an aphorism, often containing a divine revelation; literally a 'thread'.

Swadhisthana: the second **chakra**, at the genitals.

tamas: the *guna* (quality) of darkness and inertia.

Tantra: a manual; a text describing Tantric beliefs and practices; a spiritual path aimed at the achievement of *moksha* through such techniques as meditation, **mantra** and *maithuna*.

Taoism: the Chinese 'Way' described in ancient texts such as the *Tao Te Ching* and containing sexual elements akin to **Tantra**.

tiravam: female ejaculate.

tri-kona: downward-pointing triangle; pubic triangle; symbol of the emanation of the universe.

tummo: a Tibetan meditation that raises the temperature of the body.

Upanishads: Indian scriptures.

Vajrayana: the Buddhist form of **Tantra**.

vajroli mudra: sucking up fluids from the vagina into the penis; an exercise to strengthen the sexual muscles.

Veda: ancient Sanskrit hymns and legends.

Vedanta: a school of philosophy; literally translated as 'the end of knowledge'; the culmination of the *Veda*.

velli: silver (i.e. semen – compare with *pon*).

vintu: semen.

vira: a *sadhaka* (Tantric devotee) who has reached a high level; virile hero.

Vishuddhi: the fifth **chakra**, at the throat.

Vishnu: one of the principal Hindu gods who can also appear in other incarnations such as **Krishna** and Rama (alternative spelling – Visnu).

whole body orgasm: ecstatic sensations that involve the entire body, not just the genitals.

yantra: a geometric diagram of an energy field, used in meditation.

yoga: union of the individual soul with the Absolute.

yogin: a man following the path of *Yoga*.

yogini: female partner in Tantric sex; semi-divine beings who inhabit the bodies of women during sex; a woman following the path of **yoga**.

yogini-vaktra: 'mouth of the *yogini*'; vulva.

yoni: Sanskrit for a woman's genitals; vulva, vagina, womb or all three together.

yonimani: clitoris.

yonipuja: worship of the vulva.

yonitattva: vulval essence; sexual fluid from the vagina.

Taking it further

Further reading

In India, many laugh at what they call the 'textbook Tantrikas' – that's to say, Westerners who learn from books. Well, yes, devoting several years of your life to studying in India with a genuine guru would undoubtedly be a better way. But if you don't have several years or don't wish to live in India, the books below will very quickly provide you with a comprehensive understanding of the subject. The practical side is then up to you.

Avalon, Arthur, *Mahanirvana Tantra of the Great Liberation* (Kessinger Publishing Co., 2004).

The *Mahanirvana Tantra* or, to give it its English title, *Tantra of the Great Liberation*, is regarded as Sir John Woodroffe/Arthur Avalon's most important translation. The *Tantra* was first published in Bengali in 1876 and an 'inaccurate version' – according to Woodroffe – appeared in English in Calcutta around the turn of the century. He determined to set the record straight. His real reason for selecting it, however, was probably that it presented a relatively 'safe' version of Tantra, acceptable to intellectual Hindus and the least likely to cause offence in Britain. He admitted as much in his Preface: 'This Tantra is, further, one which is well known and esteemed,' he wrote, 'though perhaps more highly so amongst that portion of the Indian public which favours 'reformed' Hinduism than amongst some Tantrikas, to whom, as I have been told, certain of its provisions appear to display unnecessary timidity.' Clearly, Woodroffe wanted to distance himself from those 'Tantrikas' as if he himself had no contact with them. Nevertheless, this is an important chance to read an actual Tantra rather than just a book about Tantra.

Avalon, Arthur, *The Serpent Power: Secrets of Tantric and Shaktic Yoga* (Dover Publications, 1976).

This is the most famous of the books by Sir John Woodroffe, writing under the pseudonym of Arthur Avalon. The serpent is, of course, *Kundalini*, the energy that Tantrikas believe lies coiled at the base of the spine, and this is the book that did so much to introduce the concept to the West. Most of the book is taken up with Woodroffe's lengthy and learned Introduction which is followed by translations of two Tantras. Not an easy read but invaluable for those who seek a deeper understanding.

Douglas, Nik, *Sexual Secrets: The Alchemy of Ecstasy* (Inner Traditions Bear and Co., 1999).

Douglas, Nik, *Spiritual Sex: Secrets of Tantra from Ice Age to the New Millennium* (Pocket Books, 1998).

Nik Douglas is an authority on *Tantra*, having spent years travelling in India, Sri Lanka, Nepal, Sikkim, Thailand and Indonesia and studying with such figures as Ajit Mookerjee, Durga Das Shastri, Dudjom Rinpoche and Gangotri Giri. His film *Tantra: Indian Rites of Ecstasy* was produced by Mick Jagger and Robert Fraser and includes footage of a sex ritual at the cremation ground at Tarapith. The first of these two books seeks out the roots of Tantra in prehistoric times and follows the development of the beliefs and techniques up to the modern era. It's a serious book for those with a genuine interest in the subject. The second title is a bestseller and covers technique in detail.

Dupuche, John R. (trans.), *The Kula Ritual, As Elaborated in Chapter 29 of the Tantraloka* (Abhinavagupta, Motilal Banarsidass Publishers, 2006).

This fascinating insight into the mindset and practices of authentic Tantrikas was written by the sage Abhinavagupta in the tenth century. Chapter 29 is the one that details the sexualized rituals, but anyone looking for erotic stimulation will be disappointed on several grounds. In the first place, the language is extremely obscure and even the explanatory commentary added by the guru Jayaratha in the thirteenth century adds little clarity. Secondly, this translation by John R. Dupuche sticks so literally to the original text that it needs a further translation into plain English itself. So this is an important book but one for the true scholar of Tantra, rather than the casual practitioner.

Feuerstein, Georg, *Sacred Sexuality* (Inner Traditions, 1992).

A stimulating account of sacred sex throughout history all over the world.

Gordon White, David, *Kiss of the Yogini* (University of Chicago Press, 2003).

An alluring title for a scholarly book that is also readable. David Gordon White, a professor of religious studies at the University of California, convincingly demonstrates that in early South Asian Tantra it was not the sex but the sexual fluids that were considered to have transformative and magical properties. The book includes the first English translations of passages from more than a dozen important Tantras.

Gordon White, David (ed.), *Tantra in Practice* (Princeton University Press, 2000).

This book brings together 36 essays on various aspects of Tantra. There's very little about sex but plenty for those who would like to understand Tantra in a wider context

Mookerjee, Ajit, *Kundalini: The Arousal of the Inner Energy* (Thames and Hudson, 1982).

Mookerjee, Ajit, *Kali: The Feminine Force* (Thames and Hudson, 1988).

Mookerjee, Ajit, and Khanna, Madhu, *The Tantric Way* (New York Graphic Society, 1977 and Thames and Hudson, 1989).

Ajit Mookerjee (1915–90) was at one time director and curator of the Crafts Museum in New Delhi, and an enthusiastic collector of Tantric art. Nik Douglas (see p. 264) recounts how, when he was once visiting Mookerjee's house, a *sadhu* woman (a woman who has renounced all material things) arrived and began abusing Mookerjee. Mookerjee prostrated himself before her, garlanded her with flowers and explained that she was a living goddess...and his ex-wife. The first of the above books explains that attitude, for Kali was the 'terrible goddess' but a goddess nevertheless. The second is an excellent explanation of *Kundalini* while the third is a detailed explanation of the theory of Tantra. All Mookerjee's books are highly authoritative but also colourful and readable.

Mumford, Dr Jonn, *Ecstasy Through Tantra* (Llewellyn, 1988).

Dr Jonn Mumford, also known as Swami Anandakapila Saraswati, wrote his first book, *Psychosomatic Yoga*, in 1961 and has been a significant force in the development of Tantra in the West ever since. A man who straddles East and West, he is reputed to be able to slow his heartbeat to almost nothing, hold his breath for over five minutes and stop and start bleeding. This is a book for those who are interested in the 'sex magick' aspect of Tantra. His other books include *The Chakra and Kundalini Workbook, The Karma Manual* and *Death: Beginning or End?*

Pandit, M.P., *Kundalini Yoga: A Brief Study of Sir John Woodroffe's 'The Serpent Power'* (India: Motilal Banarsidass, 2002).

For a critique of *The Serpent Power*, read this assessment by M.P. Pandit.

Rawson, Philip, *The Art of Tantra* (Thames and Hudson, 1973).

In 1971, Philip Rawson, as Dean of the School of Art and Design at Goldsmith's College, University of London, organized the first comprehensive exhibition of Tantric art at the Hayward Gallery. This book is based upon the catalogue he wrote at the time. It is possibly the most exhilarating account of Tantric sex that has ever been written, and the numerous colour and black and white illustrations are inspiring.

Van Lysebeth, André, *Tantra: The Cult of the Feminine* (Weiser Books, 1995).

If you're going to buy just one more serious book about Tantric sex then the choice is between this and Nik Douglas's *Spiritual Sex*. Here in a single volume you have the history of Tantric sex, the philosophy and the modern practice.

Versluis, Arthur, *The Secret History of Western Sexual Mysticism* (Destiny Books, 2008).

A short, easy read which makes clear that the West, too, has had its own versions of 'Tantric sex' going back to Greek and Roman antiquity and beyond.

Woodroffe, Sir John, *The Great Liberation* (India: Nesma Books, 2001).

Woodroffe, Sir John, *Tantra and Bengal: An Indian Soul in a European Body?* (Kathleen Taylor, Routledge Curzon, 2001).

Sir John Woodroffe was the British High Court Judge who played a key role in bringing Tantra to the West. He wrote as the mystical 'Arthur Avalon', a pseudonym which, as he readily admitted, covered not just himself but also various Indian scholars, including his close friend A.B. Ghose. Probably his best-known book is *The Serpent Power* which spread knowledge of *Kundalini Yoga* in the West. This biography is in two parts; the first part focuses on Woodroffe's life in Calcutta at the beginning of the twentieth century and the second part is an assessment of his handling of his subject and his contribution to Western understanding of Tantra.

Tantric sex and the Internet

If you put 'Tantric sex' into your search engine you'll find thousands of sites. Very few, however, have any connection with the real thing. The following sites will all expand your knowledge of authentic Tantra, its sexualized rites and modern adaptations for Western couples.

www.shivashakti.com

A very serious and comprehensive resource. It includes translations of Tantras and other important texts, information about all aspects of authentic Tantra, and useful links.

www.religiousworlds.com/mandalam/index.html
American mirror site for shivashakti.com

www.tantraworks.com

A useful site from author Nik Douglas (see Further reading) with excellent links and brief articles on a range of Tantra subjects including art, temples, ancient Tantra and modern versions.

www.sacred-texts.com

An excellent website that contains all the great sacred texts of the world. As far as Tantra is concerned, you can read Sir John Woodroffe's translation of the *Mahanirvana Tantra* (see p. 263), together with his hugely detailed Introduction, as well as several of his essays on the subject. None of what he wrote is easy going and, writing at the beginning of the twentieth century, he was extremely cautious about sex. Nevertheless, anyone who has a serious interest will get more out of this than many more recent works.

www.asiatica.org/publications/ijts/

The by-subscription International Journal of Tantric Studies online. Very learned articles about the history of Tantra, its diverse forms and its practitioners.

Choosing workshops and courses

There is no formal qualification for a guru. Thus there are such sayings as 'when the moment is right the guru appears' and 'you'll know your guru when you meet him.' Normally, someone would become a guru after years of study under an existing guru, the teachings and procedures being handed on in a process going back to, perhaps, the seventh century. But if I choose to call myself a Tantric sex guru, no-one can stop me. Many people do just that, in India as much as in the West, without any proper knowledge of Tantra.

Most workshops in the West teach 'neo-*Tantra*' which has very little to do with the authentic sexualized rituals and beliefs, but there are gurus in the West who lead *cakras* (circles or groups) in the original Oriental style of Tantra. And, of course, the Eastern and Western styles can themselves take various different forms. So the first thing to do is to find out precisely what style of Tantric sex is being taught and what you'll be expected to do. Some workshops are 'clothes on' and you'll only practise intimate techniques in the privacy of your own room. At the other extreme are courses where students will, at some stage, explore sacred sex in the company of others or even with different partners. If a course is to be any good, it should be taking you further than you've ever been before but be certain before you sign up that it's not taking you too far beyond your present comfort zone or into areas which, for you, could result in the complete opposite of bliss.

Find out something about the credentials of the people leading the course. Ask who they studied with, find out how many courses they've already led and see if you can get any testimonials. After you've spoken to them ask yourself this: 'Do these people sound as if they've reached a higher level?' If you're taking a course close to where you live you may not be risking a lot of money but if you're contemplating flying somewhere for several days, the outlay could be significant so you're entitled to ask questions. If the course seems unreasonably expensive and its leaders overly eager to receive your deposit, then you may feel they haven't themselves reached the higher state to which you yourself aspire. However, it's not just an issue of money. You could be setting yourself up for psychological and relationship problems if your teachers don't really know what they're doing. If you sign up for 'Tantric sex' then sex, in some form or another, is what you're going to get. But in the traditional system, before the power of sex was unleashed, you first had to demonstrate that you had attained a certain emotional and spiritual level. 'Beginners' (*pashus*) weren't allowed to take part in Tantric sex. On many modern courses that safeguard doesn't apply. If you're a stable person there's probably no risk, but if you're a person with issues from your past, a course could unleash unexpected forces. I'm not going to recommend any particular courses because to do that in a fair way I would have had to have been on all of them. Just remember that anybody can set themselves up as an expert on Tantra. Be cautious and do your research.

Appendix I: How Tantra came to the West

In 1591, three ships sailed from England around the Cape of Good Hope to the Arabian Sea, the first of many that were to bring back cotton, silk, indigo, tea, saltpetre – and, in time, Tantric sex.

Of course, people in India were not the only ones to have noticed that, in addition to being highly pleasurable, sexual intercourse could create altered states of consciousness. The ancient Egyptians certainly had a kind of sacred sex, as did the Sumerians. The Greeks and Romans had their 'Mystery' traditions and their *hieros gamos* or sacred marriage to a deity. And there had even been early Christian groups, like the Carpocratians who argued that, just as God had made sunlight available to all, so He had sexual pleasure. But essentially, news of Tantric sex arrived almost in the way of a revolutionary call-to-arms, inspiring small 'cells' of people to get together and dare to cast off the yoke of guilt.

Some historians argue that sexual mysticism continued to be part of Christian religious life in Europe right through from antiquity without interruption. But the evidence is thin. The so-called Sheela-na-Gigs which adorn some Norman churches of Romanesque design are not, in my opinion, akin to Tantric images of goddesses displaying their *yonis* but are, given their generally grotesque proportions, warnings *against* lust. When the occasional preachers and practitioners of 'mystical sex' came to the notice of the authorities, like the German Buttlar circle – the main members of which were tortured by the government in 1706 – the normal reaction was suppression, not tolerance.

It was the Kabbalah, an esoteric aspect of Judaism, which kept sexual mysticism alive in Europe through texts such as the thirteenth century *Zohar*. The *Zohar* taught that sexual union not only increases the reservoir of peace on Earth but brings pleasure to the feminine aspect of the Divine, the *shekinah*. Throughout the eighteenth century, as employees of the East India Company were returning with their tales of exotic sexual rites, there were eager groups of intellectuals, artists and religious pioneers who had already been prepared, as it were, by their delving into the secrets of the Kabbalah. They included, crucially, Emanuel Swedenborg (1688–1772), the Swedish mystic and scientist, and Count Nicolaus von Zinzendorf (1700–60), leader of the Moravian Church, the first Protestant Church, which, having been persecuted in its homeland, set up in a Chapel in London's Fetter Lane in 1738. There, for a period of a few years, the congregation followed practices that were increasingly Kabbalistic and Tantric in character, with all night 'love feasts' and images of couples drawn inside vulvas. One woman, applying for permanent membership of the Chapel, wrote how at the 'love feast our Saviour was pleased to make me Suck his wounds' a reference to the Moravian's then view of Christ's side-wound as a symbolic vulva. Her name was Catherine Armitage and she was to become the mother of one of the greatest artists of the spiritual and erotic, William Blake (1757–1827).

By the middle of the nineteenth century, a quasi-Tantric commune was established in New York. This was the Oneida Community which practised 'complex marriage' or free love using male continence. In other words, the men didn't ejaculate. Each woman had an average of three partners a week and, in an age before efficient birth control, male continence was a way of trying to prevent the women from all becoming pregnant. It also, of course, allowed the men to have almost unlimited sexual encounters.

However there were others for whom the spiritual aspect of 'male continence' was all important. One of those was a gynaecologist from Chicago called Alice Bunker-Stockham who, having travelled to India, saw that Tantra could have benefits for Westerners. She didn't accept Tantra entirely but invented her own version which she called Karezza after the Italian word *carezza*, meaning 'caress'. It's a fairly apt title because, during intercourse, she recommended couples do just that, and little more. Stockham said she experienced powerful spiritual feelings using this method. Karezza isn't Tantric sex, but the parallels are obvious.

Britain's answer to Alice Stockham was Marie Stopes who started the birth control clinics that continue to this day and who wrote a beautiful book called *Married Love*, first published in 1918. Stopes contribution to Western Tantra was her opposition to coitus interruptus (in which a man withdraws just before climax and ejaculates outside the vagina) because it prevented a woman absorbing a man's 'secretions'. In her book she wrote that a man shouldn't ejaculate frequently because 'all the vital energy and nerve force' as well as the 'precious chemical substances' could then be retained for other 'creative' things. This, of course, accords with Tantra, particularly the Buddhist school.

Meanwhile, a man who went under the mystical name of Arthur Avalon was intent on promoting not a Westernized version of Tantra, but real Indian Tantra. He was probably the first true Western scholar of Tantra, especially Shakta Tantra which worshipped the 'Supreme Deity' as female. He wrote several books on the subject of which the most famous is *The Serpent Power* (see Taking it further). In fact, he did somewhat play down the sexual aspects of Tantra but that's hardly surprising given that his real name was Sir John Woodroffe and that he became Advocate General of Bengal and, in 1915, Chief Justice of the High Court of India at Calcutta. Or, rather, he didn't so much play it down as bury it under an avalanche of scholarship which made his books extremely difficult to read. Although he was extremely prolific, his books didn't, therefore, have much impact outside intellectual circles.

Probably the first person to get through to large numbers of people in the West was an Indian guru in a beanie who went under the name Bhagwan Shree Rajneesh, and later Osho. During the 1960s he made a series of speeches promoting Tantra which the Western press vilified as advocating 'free love'. Which, in fact, he did. His speeches were later compiled under the title *From Sex to*

Superconsciousness. Rajneesh said that: 'For Tantra everything is holy, nothing is unholy.' Sex, he argued, had to be thoroughly experienced if it was to be transcended. In fact, Tantra was only one of the many belief systems that he drew on, but it's the one for which he's remembered – along with the various scandals that rocked the community he set up in Wasco County, Oregon in 1981 (including a 'salmonella attack' on local restaurants and a plot to assassinate the U.S. Attorney for Oregon).

Because of those scandals, Tantrikas don't tend to mention Rajneesh much these days, but he had given Tantric sex a new direction suitable for most Westerners, and which should really be called neo-Tantra. Neo-Tantra, as taught by 'gurus' such as Margot Anand, author of *The Art of Sexual Ecstasy,* stresses lengthy, spiritual lovemaking but otherwise has little to do with the real thing.

Index

Image credits